INTRODUCTION
TO
PHARMACEUTICS-II

(According to P.C.I. Education Regulation – 1991)

FOURTH EDITION

INTRODUCTION TO PHARMACEUTICS-II

(According to P.C.I. Education Regulation – 1991)

FOURTH EDITION

ASHOK K. GUPTA
M. Pharm (Pharmaceutics)
Head of Department, Pharmacy,
Govt. Polytechnic for Women, Chandigarh

and

S.S. BAJAJ
M. Pharm, LL.B.
Ex. Head of Department, Pharmacy,
Govt. Polytechnic for Women, Chandigarh

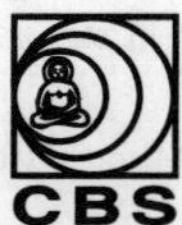

CBS Publishers & Distributors Pvt Ltd

New Delhi • Bengaluru Chennai Kochi Kolkata Lucknow Mumbai
Hyderabad Jharkhand Nagpur Patna Pune Uttarakhand

Introduction to
Pharmaceutics II
(According to PCI Education Regulation, 1991)
Fourth Edition

ISBN-13: 978-81-239-0339-2
ISBN-10: 81-239-0339-1

Fourth Edition: 2000
Reprint: 2001, 2002, 2003, 2004, 2005, 2006, 2007, 2008, 2009, 2011, 2013, 2015, 2016, 2017, 2018, 2019, 2022, 2023, **2025**
First Edition: 1986
Second Edition: 1987
Third Edition: 1994

Published by **Satish Kumar Jain** and produced by **Varun Jain** for

CBS Publishers & Distributors Pvt Ltd
4819/XI Prahlad Street, 24 Ansari Road, Daryaganj, New Delhi 110 002, India.
Ph: 011-23266838, 23289259 Website: www.cbspd.com
e-mail: delhi@cbspd.com

Corporate Office: 204 FIE, Industrial Area, Patparganj, Delhi 110 092
Ph: 011-4934 4934 Fax: 011-4934 4935
e-mail: publishing@cbspd.com; publicity@cbspd.com

Branches

- **Bengaluru:** Seema House 2975, 17th Cross, KR Road, Banasankari 2nd Stage, Bengaluru 560 070, Karnataka, India
  Ph: +91-80-26771678/79 Fax: +91-80-26771680 e-mail: bangalore@cbspd.com
- **Chennai:** 7, Subbaraya Street, Shenoy Nagar, Chennai 600 030, Tamil Nadu, India
  Ph: +91-44-26680620, 26681266 Fax: +91-44-42032115 e-mail: chennai@cbspd.com
- **Kochi:** 42/1325, 1326, Power House Road, Opp KSEB, Power House, Ernakulum Kochi 682 018, Kerala, India
  Ph: +91-484-4059061-65,67 Fax: +91-484-4059065 e-mail: kochi@cbspd.com
- **Kolkata:** 147, Hind Ceramics Compound, 1st Floor, Nilgunj Road, Belghoria, Kolkata-700056, West Bengal, India
  Ph: +033-25633055, 033-25633056 e-mail: kolkata@cbspd.com
- **Lucknow:** Basement, Khushnuma Complex, 7 Meerabai Marg (Behind Jawahar Bhawan), Lucknow-226001, UP, India
  Ph: +0522-4000032 e-mail: tiwari.lucknow@cbspd.com
- **Mumbai:** PWD Shed, Gala no 25/26, Ramchandra Bhatt Marg, Next to JJ Hospital Gate no. 2, Opp. Union Bank of India, Noorbaug, Mumbai-400009, Maharashtra, India
  Ph: 022-66661880/89 e-mail: mumbai@cbspd.com

Representatives

- Hyderabad 0-9885175004
- Jharkhand 0-9811541605
- Nagpur 0-8692091830
- Patna 0-9334159340
- Pune 0-9664372571
- Uttarakhand 0-9716462459

Printed at Glorious Printers, Jhilmil Industrial Area, Delhi, India

Preface to the Fourth Edition

In recent years the pharmaceutical technology has undergone a sea change with the development of new techniques of method of preparation and testing of pharmaceuticals. With these developments pharmaceutical education has also seen many changes.

With the changing trends in pharmaceutical education at higher levels the Pharmacy Council of India according to E.R. 1991 has revised the course contents for Diploma Pharmacy students to bring their knowledge up-to-date. A number of new subjects have been introduced and lot of changes are made in the existing ones. Similarly in the subject of Pharmaceuticals II new topics on veterinary doses and dental and cosmetic preparations are introduced. The authors have tried their best to cover all the topics according to the syllabus prescribed by Pharmacy Council of India in a very simple language. Wherever necessary the subject matter is illustrated by suitable diagrams.

As the previous editions were warmly accepted by the teachers and the students all over the country, this edition will create more interest as it covers the whole syllabus and in a precise and systematic way and will meet all the needs and requirements of the teachers as well as the students of pharmacy.

In the present edition, exhaustive revision questions in the form of very short answer type questions, fill in the blanks, short answer type questions on the pattern of (VARIOUS EXAMINING BODIES OF DIFFERENT STATES) have been introduced at the end of each chapter. They will help the students by revising these questions themselves and help them to secure very good marks in the examination.

Our sincere thanks are due to all teachers and students who have appreciated the previous editions and sent their criticism and suggestions to bring the present edition upto everyone's expectations. Suggestions and comments for further improvement of the book will be appreciated and acknowledged.

We express our sincere gratitude to Sh. Satish Kumar Jain and Sh. Vinod Kumar Jain for their keen interest and painstaking efforts in bringing out the present edition of this book in a short span of time.

May, 2000 ASHOK K. GUPTA

Contents

1

Prescription

Prescription is an order written by a physician, dentist or any other registered medical practitioner to a pharmacist to compound and dispense a specific medication for the patient. The order is accompanied by directions for the pharmacist that what type of preparation is to be prepared and how much is to be prepared. It is also accompanied with the directions for the patient that how much medicament is to be taken, how many times it is to be taken or at what time and how it is to be taken.

The prescription provides a common link of mutual interest between the physician, the pharmacist and the patient. It is the duty of the pharmacist to serve the medication needs of the patient according to the intention of the prescriber. It is not sufficient that the pharmacist should only compound the specific medication but he should make the patient understand about the proper administration of the drug and ensure that the patient sticks to these instructions. At the same time the pharmacist must maintain and respect the confidentiality of both the physician regarding the treatment given as well as that of the patient regarding the nature of his illness and the medication taken by him.

The prescriptions are generally written in the language of the area in which they originate but Latin words are frequently used in the prescription writing because in the olden days the medicines were written in Latin language which was understood all over the world. Still the use of Latin abbreviations in the prescription writing is very common, specially in dosage instructions.

PARTS OF A PRESCRIPTION

A complete prescription should have the following parts :

1. Date
2. Name, age, sex and address of the patient
3. Superscription
4. Inscription
5. Subscription
6. Signatura
7. Signature, address and registration number of prescriber.

1. Date

Date must be written on the prescription by the prescriber at the same time when it is written. The date on the prescription helps a pharmacist to find out the cases where prescription is brought for dispensing long time after its issue. Prescriptions containing narcotic or other habit-forming drugs must bear the date. The prescriptions should be filled within a reasonable time after it is written. If the prescription is brought for filling after two or three days from the date when it was written then the pharmacist must question if the intention of the prescriber and the needs of the patient can still be met.

2. Name, Age, Sex, and Address of the Patient

Name, age, sex, and address of the patient must be written on the prescription. If it is not written then the pharmacist himself should ask the patient about these particulars and put down at the top of the prescription. This avoids the possibility of giving the finished product to a person other than the one it is meant for. Patient's full name must be written instead of surname or the family name.

Age and sex of the patient specially in the case of children helps the pharmacist in checking the medication and the dose. Therefore there will be less danger of its being administered to the wrong member of the family or the hospital ward having similar names. The address of the patient is recorded to help for any reference at a later stage, to contact the patient or to deliver the medication personally.

3. Superscription

The superscription is represented by a symbol Rx which is always written at the beginning of the prescription. In the days of mythology and superstition the symbol was considered as a prayer to Jupiter, the God of healing, for quick recovery of the patient but now this symbol is understood as an abbreviation of the Latin word recipe, meaning "take thou" or "you take".

4. Inscription

This is the main part of the prescription. It contains the names and quantities of the prescribed ingredients. The names of the ingredients are written each on a separate line, followed by the quantity ordered and the last item written is generally the vehicle or diluent. In complex prescriptions containing several ingredients the inscription is divided into three parts (a) the base or the active medicament which is intended to produce the therapeutic effect; (b) the adjuvant which is included either to enhance the action of the medicament or to make the product more palatable; (c) the vehicle which is either used to dissolve the solid substances and/or to increase the volume of the preparation for ease of administration.

Now a days only a few prescriptions are compounded by pharmacists. A majority of prescriptions are written for medications already prepared into dosage forms by industrial manufacturers. The pharmacists are only required to dispense the ready-made dosage form of drugs which has eliminated the compounding of prescriptions.

5. Subscription

This part of the prescription contains prescriber's directions to the pharmacist regarding the dosage form to be prepared and number of doses to be dispensed. Since now-a-days only a few prescriptions are compounded therefore such directions are less frequent.

6. Signatura

It is usually abbreviated as "Sig" on the prescriptions and consists of the directions to be given to the patient regarding the administration of the drug. It usually indicates the quantity of medicament or number or dosage units to be taken, how many times in a day or at what time it should be taken and the manner in which it is to be administered or applied. These instructions must be transferred to the label of the container in which the medicament is to be dispensed and ensure that the patient follows these instructions carefully.

7. Signature, Address and Registration Number of the Prescriber

All other parts of the prescription may be printed or type-written but the prescriber's name must be hand-written and should be signed with ink. This eliminates the danger of dispensing medicament on a spurious order and it authenticates the prescription. The prescriptions containing narcotic or other habit-forming drugs must bear the address and registration number of the prescriber. This identifies the special licence which a prescriber must have to prescribe the narcotic and other habit-forming drugs.

Handling of Prescription

1. Receiving
2. Reading and checking
3. Collecting the materials
4. Weighing
5. Compounding
6. Finishing.

1. Receiving

The prescription should be received from the patient by the pharmacist himself. Under no circumstances an unauthorised person should try to receive or read the prescription.

An Example of a Typical Prescription

General Hospital

Date	21.6.86
Name	Sh. Raman Kumar
Age	40 years
Sex	Male
Address	817, Sector-20 Chandigarh

Rx (Superscription)

Potassium Bromide	8 gm	(Inscription)
Tincture Nux Vomica	8 ml	
Chloroform Water q.s.	120 ml	

Fiat mistura (Subscription)

Sig. Cochleare magnum ter in die post cibos sumenda. (Signatura)

(Signature of the Prescriber)

S.C. Aggarwal M.D.

Regd. No. 10234

2. Reading and Checking

A brief examination of each prescription should be made immediately upon receiving it from the patient. This will tell the pharmacist about the nature of the dosage form to be prepared and he can estimate the time required for preparing it. If a long time is needed for compounding the prescription then he must tell the patient about the time required for filling the prescription so that he may wait or return after some time. In some cases the patient's name, age and address may not be written on the prescription, in such cases these informations should be enquired from the patient and put down on the prescription.

Careful examination of the prescription should be made only behind the counter, so that if there is any doubt regarding the prescription ingredients or directions or there in any error in writing the prescription, the patient should not come to know about it. If there is any doubt the pharmacist should consult the other pharmacists or the prescriber.

Every prescription should be read and understood completely before compounding it. Every word and abbreviation must be interpreted correctly. He should never guess about the meaning of an illegible or confusing word. It may lead to serious consequences. If there is any doubt he should consult the fellow pharmacists or the prescriber.

As the number of drugs available in the market are increasing, the mistakes, due to the similarity or pronunciation and spellings are also increasing. In such cases a pharmacist has to take a great care specially when the prescriptions are received orally. Examples of such drugs which look alike or sound alike are given below :

Apresoline	Priscoline
Compocillin	Ampicillin
Daricon	Darvon
Digoxin	Digitoxin
Indocin	Lincocin
Prednisone	Prednisolone
Qinine	Quinidine

Before the start of compounding the prescription, the pharmacist must ensure that what he is going to do and what type of finished product he will obtain.

3. Collecting and Weighing the Materials

Materials to be used in compounding the prescription should be collected on the left hand side of the balance and arranged in the order in which they are to be mixed. The materials which are weighed should be shifted to right hand side of the balance. This gives a mechanical check of ingredients which has been weighed. The label on every stock bottle should be read at least three times :

(a) When taken from the shelf or drawer.
(b) When the contents are removed for weighing or measuring.
(c) When the containers are returned back to its proper place.

4. Compounding

This is the most important phase in handling the prescription. In this case proper drug is dispensed in a suitable form. This can be achieved only if accuracy, cleanliness and proper techniques are observed in the preparation of any medication. Only one prescription should be compounded at one time. If two or more prescriptions are dispensed at the same time, one is likely to make serious mistakes by dispensing wrong drugs. Attention should not be diverted by talking to friends, attending the telephone or engaging in other directions.

Now a days majority of the prescriptions are written for the pre-compounded dosage forms supplied by the pharmaceutical manufacturers which require no compounding or mixing by the pharmacist. When a prescription requiring compounding is received the pharmacist should decide the calculations, special adjuvants and order of mixing then he should proceed further as described above.

5. Finishing

The compounded medicaments should be filled in suitable containers depending on the quantity of the medication to be dispensed and the method of its use. Various types of containers used in pharmacy are : round vials used for filling the unit dosage forms such as tablets and capsules; oval prescription bottles used for filling liquids of low viscosity; wide mouth bottles used for filling the liquids of high viscosity, large quantities of tablets or capsules and bulk powders; ointment jars and collapsible tubes used for filling the ointments, creams or semisolid dosage forms; dropper bottles used for dispensing the eye drops, ear drops or other liquids to be administered by drops; sifter top containers used for dispensing the powders meant to be applied externally by sprinkling etc. The container should be selected approximately of the same volume as that of the medication to be dispensed.

Most of the containers are available in various sizes, shapes, colours and compositions. They may be made up of glass, plastic or suitable metal. Most of the glass containers are made from colourless or amber coloured glass. The latter being used for dispensing light sensitive medications. Plastic containers and collapsible tubes are also widely used for dispensing various types of dosage forms.

The filled containers are suitably labelled. A good quality of paper and adhesive should be used for labelling the containers. The size of the label should be proportional to the size of the container and should be neatly hand-written or preferably typed. The following information should be written on all labels :

1. Name of the prescription
2. Name of the patient, age and sex
3. Registration number
4. Date of dispensing
5. Directions for its use
6. Expiry date, if any
7. Storage conditions
8. Name and address of the pharmacy.

The label should be placed almost in the centre leaving equal space from the bottom and top of the bottle. On collapsible tubes it should be placed near the top to avoid concealment and wrinkling as the tube is rolled up from the bottom during its use. Special adhesives should be used for fixing the labels on the collapsible tubes.

Some containers like ophthalmic ointment tubes, eye drop and ear drop bottles and other small containers which lack sufficient surface area for attaching the label may be labelled with the serial number and packed in bigger container which is properly labelled. Special directions like "For external use only." and "Shake the bottle before use." must be attached to the bottle as secondary label.

After preparing and labelling, the compounded prescription should be thoroughly examined to ensure accuracy, quality and safety of the prescription. The checker should first check the written prescription and then the contents of the container for colour, odour or any other indication for the correctness and quality of the medication. If the checker finds that the compounded prescription is correct then he must put his signatures on the prescription. Before the prescription is handed over to the patient the container must be thoroughly polished so as to remove the finger prints.

Latin Terms and Abbreviations Commonly Used in Prescription Writing

Latin term or phrase	*Abbreviation*	*English meaning*
Ad	ad.	to, up to
Ad libitum	ad. lib.	at pleasure, as desired
Admove	admov.	apply
Agita	agit.	shake, stir
Alter	alt.	the other, alternate
Alternis horis	alt. hrs.	alternate hours
Ana	a a.	of each
Ante	a.	before
Ante cibos	a.c.	before meals
Applicandus	applicand	to be applied
Aqua	aq.	water
Aqua bulliens	aq. bull.	boiling water
Aqua destillata	aq. dest.	distilled water
Auris dextra	a.d.	right ear
Auris laeva	a.l.	left ear
Auristillae	auristill	ear drops
Bis in die	b.i.d.	twice a day
Capsula	caps.	capsule
Capiat	cap.	let him take
Capiendus	capiend.	to be taken
Cataplasma	cataplasm	poultice
Charta	chart.	powder, powder paper
Cibos	cibos.	food, meals
Cochleare amplum / magnum / maximum	coch amp. / mag. / max.	one tablespoonful
Cochleare medium / modicum	coch med. / mod.	one desertspoonful
Cochleare minimum / parvum	coch min. / parv.	one teaspoonful
Collunarium	collunar.	a nose wash

Latin term or phrase	*Abbreviation*	*English meaning*
Collutorium	collut.	a mouth wash
Collyrium	collyr.	an eye wash
Congius	cong; c	a gallon
Cum	c	with
Cum duplo	c. dup.	with twice as much
Cum parte aequale	c. pt. aeq.	with an equal quantity
Cyathus	cyath.	a glass
Dentur	dent.	give, let it be given
Dexter	dext.	right
Diebus alternis	dieb. alt.	every other day
Divide	div.	divide
Dolore urgente	dol. urg.	when the pain is severe
Emulsio	emul.	an emulsion
E	—	with
E. lacte	e. lact.	with milk
Ex. aqua	ex. aq.	with water
Ex. modo prescripto	e.m.p.	in the manner prescribed
Fiat, fit, fiant.	ft.	make, let it be made
Granum, grana	gr.	a grain
Gutta, guttae	gtt.	a drop, drops
Hac nocte	hac noct.	to night
Hora	h.	an hour
Hora somni	h.s.	at bed time
In dies	In. d.	daily
Inter cibos	i.c.	during meals
Injectio	Inj.	an injection
Laevo	l.	left
Levis	lev.	light
Linimentum	lin.	a liniment
Liquor	liq.	solution
Mane	m.	morning
Minimum	min.	a minim
Misce	m.	mix, let (it) be mixed
Mistura	mist.	a mixture
Mitte	mitt.	send
Mitte tales	mitt tal.	send such
Modo dicto	m. dict.	as directed, as stated
Modo prescripto	m. pres.	as prescribed
More dicto	m. dict.	in the manner prescribed

Latin term or phrase	*Abbreviation*	*English meaning*
Nebula	nebul.	a spray
Nocte maneque	noct. maneq.	night and morning
Non repetatur	non rep, n.r.	do not repeat
Octarius	o.	a pint
Oculo utro	o.u.	each eye
Oculus dexter	o.d.	right eye
Oculus laevus	o.l.	left eye
Oculus sinister	o.s.	left eye
Omni	omn.	every
Omni hora	omn. hor, o.h.	every hour
Omni quadranta hora	omn. quadr. hor	every quarter of an hour
Omni quarta hora	omn. 4 hrs.	every four hours
Omni secunda hora	omn. 2 hrs.	every two hours
Omni mane	o.m.	every morning
Omni nocte	o.n.	every night
Os, oris	o.s.	mouth
Parti affecti applicandus	p.a.a.	to be applied to the affected part
Per os	p.o.	orally by mouth
Phiala prius agitata	p.p.a.	the bottle, being first shaken (i.e., attach a "Shake the bottle." label)
Post cibos	p.c.	after meals
Pro oculo laevo	p.o.l.	for the left eye
Pro dosi	—	as a dose
Pro re nata	p.r.n.	when necessary, occasionally
Pulvis	pulv	powder
Quantum sufficiat	q.s.	as much as sufficient
Quaque quarta hora	q.q.h.	every fourth hour
Quarter in die	q.i.d.	four times a day
Quotidie	quot.	Daily
Recipe	Rx	take
Secundum artum	s.a.	according to the art
Semis, Semi	ss.	half
Signa, signetur	sig.	write
Si opus sit	s.o.s.	when necessary
Solve	—	dissolve
Solutio	sol.	a solution
Statim	stat.	immediately

Latin term or phrase	*Abbreviation*	*English meaning*
Sumendus	sum.	to be taken
Suppositorium	supp.	a suppository
Tabella, tabletta	tab.	a tablet
Talis, tales	tal.	such
Ter in die	t.i.d.	three times a day
Ter quotidie	—	three times daily
Tussi urgente	tuss. urg.	when the cough is troublesome
Uncia	—	an ounce
Unguentum	ung.	an ointment
Utendus	u. or utend.	to be used
Unus	i	one
Duo	ii	two
Tres	iii	three
Quatuor	iv	four
Quinque	v	five
Sex	vi	six
Septem	vii	seven
Octo	viii	eight
Novem	ix	nine
Decem	x	ten
Undecim	xi	eleven
Duodecim	xii	twelve
Quindecim	xv	fifteen

CALCULATIONS INVOLVED IN DISPENSING

Before discussing the calculations which are involved in dispensing of drugs it is very necessary to have a thorough knowledge regarding weights and measures which are used in calculations. These weights and measures are discussed as follows :

Weight

It is a measure of the gravitational force acting on a body and is directly proportional to its mass. The mass remains constant and never varies because it is based on inertia whereas weight varies slightly with change in latitude, altitude, temperature and pressure. The effect of these factors is not considered unless very accurate weighings are to be done.

Measure

It is the measurement of volume of any substance. Temperature and pressure exert their effect specially on liquids and gases. The effect of these factors is only taken into consideration when accurate preparations are to be made.

There are two systems of weights and measures (a) the imperial system (b) the metric system, with which the pharmacist must be familiar. The imperial system is an old system based on arbitrary and unrelated units, e.g., grains, drachms, ounces and gallons whereas the metric system or decimal system is based on related and rationally derived units, e.g., milligrams, grams, centimeters, meters, millilitres, litres, etc. Because of its easier calculations, greater accuracy and flexibility and use in other sciences, now a days this is the most widely used system by official agencies.

Adoption of Metric System

In 1948 a committee on weights and measures legislation was appointed by the president of the Board of Trade to review the existing weights and measures legislation and to make recommendations thereof. In 1951 the committee published a report in which it was recommended that the apothecary system (Imperial system) should be abolished and the metric system should be adopted in its place. Therefore steps were taken to abolish the use of imperial system for all dealings in drugs and medicines and its use was declared illegal in pharmacy profession. Since 31st March 1969 pharmacists were required to carry out all dispensing work in metric system.

Accordingly the first changeover to the metric system appeared in the British Pharmacopoeia and British Pharmaceutical Codex published in 1963. The doses of tablets, capsules and injections were given only in metric quantities. Weights and Measures Regulations 1964 described certain equivalents in metric units that whenever strength is prescribed in the imperial units that must be dispensed according to equivalent strength in metric units.

Though the pharmacists are required to use the metric system for dispensing the prescriptions but still a large number of physicians trained to use the imperial system prescribe the drugs in the old system and some hospitals still retain it as the local standard. Some drugs are prescribed in fractional doses (1/200, 1/150, 1/100 gr). The bottles for liquids are still manufactured to contain ounce measurements rather than milliliters.

Due to the above mentioned reasons, it is still necessary to be familiar with both the systems which are described in detail as follows :

(a) Imperial System

Imperial system is divided into two systems :

(i) Avoirdupois system
(ii) Apothecaries system.

Avoirdupois system

According to this system the standard unit for weighing is pound and all other measures of mass are derived from pound. It is represented by lb.

1 lb	= 16 oz (Avoir)	
1 lb	= 7000 grains	
1 oz	= 7000/16	= 437.5 grains

Apothecaries system

It is known as troy system. The standard weight in this system is grain.

20 grain	= 1 scruple
60 grain	= 1 drachm
480 grain	= 1 ounce (Apothe)
8 drachm	= 1 ounce (Apothe)
12 ounces (Apothe)	= 1 pound (Apothe)
5760 grain	= 1 pound (Apothe)

Abbreviations commonly used in weighing

Latin name	*Symbol*	*English name*	*Equal to*	
Granum	gr	grain	1	grain
Scrupulus	℈	scruple	20	grains
Drachma	ʒ	drachm	60	grains
Uncia	oz	ounce (Avoir)	437.5	grains
Uncia	℥	ounce (Apothe)	480	grains
Libra	lb	pound (Avoir)	7000	grains
Libra	lb	pound (Apothe)	5760	grains

Measures of Capacity

Standard units for capacity are same in avoirdupois as well as apothecaries system. The standard unit is gallon and all other measures of capacity are derived from gallon.

1 gallon	= 160 fluid ounces	
1/4th of a gallon	= 1 quart	= 40 fl. ounce
1/8th of gallon	= 1 pint	= 20 fl. ounce
1/160th of a gallon	= 1 fl. ounce	
1/8th of one fl. ounce	= 1 fl. drachm	
1/60th of one fl. drachm	= 1 minim	
1 fluid ounce	= 480 minim	
1 fluid drachm	= 480/8	= 60 minim

Abbreviations commonly used in measures of capacity

Latin name	*Symbol*	*English name*	*Equal to*
Minimum	m	minim	1 minim
Fluidrachma	ʒ	fl. drachm	60 minim
Fluidunicia	℥	fl. ounce	480 minim
Octarius	O	pint	20 fl. ounces
Congius	C	gallon	160 fl. ounces

Metric System

Standard unit of measures of mass (weight) is kilogram and all other measures of mass are derived from kilogram.

1 Kilogram (kg)	= 1000 gm	
1 Hectogram (hg)	= 100 gm	
1 Decagram (dag)	= 10 gm	
1 Gram (gm)	= 1 gm	
1 Decigram (dg)	= 0.1 gm	= 100 mg
1 Centigram (cg)	= 0.01 gm	= 10 mg
1 Milligram (mg)	= 0.001 gm	= 1 mg
1 Microgram (µg, mcg)	= 1/1000 mg	

Measures of Capacity

Standard unit for measures of capacity (volume) is litre and all other measures of capacity are derived from litre.

1 litre (lt) = 1000 millilitre (ml)

Domestic Measures

1 drop	= 1 minim	= 0.06 ml
1 tea spoonful	= 1 fl. drachm	= 4 ml
1 desert spoonful	= 2 fl. drachm	= 8 ml
1 table spoonful	= 4 fl. drachm	= 15 ml
2 table spoonful	= 1 fl. ounce	= 30 ml
1 wine glassful	= 2 fl. ounce	= 60 ml
1 tea cupful	= 4 fl. ounce	= 120 ml
1 tumblerful	= 8 fl. ounce	= 240 ml

Conversion Factors

1 grain	= 64.8 mg	= 65 mg	(for all practical purposes)
1 drop	= 1 minim	= 0.06 ml	(for all practical purposes)
1 fl. ounce	= 29.57 ml	= 30 ml	(for all practical purposes)
1 gram	= 15.43 gr	= 15 gr	(for all practical purposes)

1 milligram	= 1/65 gr	= 1/65 gr	(for all practical purposes)
1 millilitre	= 16.23 minim	= 15 m	(for all practical purposes)
1 litre	= 33.8 fl. ounce		
1 kilogram	= 2.2 pound		

CALCULATIONS

Calculations based on density

Density in defined as the mass of a substance per unit volume. It has the units of mass over volume.

Specific gravity is the ratio of the weight of a substance in air to that of an equal volume of water. It does not have any units.

In the metric system both density and specific gravity are numerically equal. The density, weight and volume of any substance can be calculated from the following equations :

$$\text{Density} = \frac{\text{weight}}{\text{volume}}$$

$$\text{Weight} = \text{density} \times \text{volume}$$

$$\text{Volume} = \frac{\text{weight}}{\text{density}}$$

If any two variables are given, the third one can be calculated.

1. Calculate the weight of 120 ml of an oil whose density is 0.9624 gm/ml.

$$\text{Weight} = \text{density} \times \text{volume}$$
$$= 0.9624 \text{ gm/ml} \times 120 \text{ ml} = 115.488 \text{ gm.}$$

2. Calculate the volume of 200 gm of glycerin. The density of glycerin is 1.25 gm/ml.

$$\text{Volume} = \frac{\text{weight}}{\text{density}}$$
$$= \frac{200 \text{ gm}}{1.25 \text{ gm/ml}} = 160 \text{ ml.}$$

3. Calculate the weight of 1 litre of alcohol whose density is 0.816 gm/ml.

$$\text{Weight} = \text{density} \times \text{volume}$$
$$= 0.816 \text{ gm/ml} \times 1000 \text{ ml} = 816 \text{ gm.}$$

Conversions from Imperial to metric and metric to Imperial systems

1. How many mg are in one grain.

Since 15.43 gr = 1 gm

$$1 \text{ gr} = \frac{1}{15.43} \text{ gm} = 0.0648 \text{ gm} = 64.8 \text{ mg}$$

$\therefore$ 1 gr = 64.8 mg.

2. How many grams are in 1 ounce (Apothe).

1 ounce (Apothe) = 480 gr

Since 15.43 gr = 1 gm

$$1 \text{ gr} = \frac{1}{15.43}$$

$$480 \text{ gr} = \frac{1}{15.43} \times 480 = 31.11 \text{ gm}$$

$\therefore$ 1 ounce (Apothe) = 31.11 gm.

3. How many grams are in 1 ounce (Avoir).

1 ounce (Avoir) = 437.5 gr

Since 15.43 gr = 1 gm

$$1 \text{ gr} = \frac{1}{15.43} \text{ gm}$$

$$437.5 \text{ gr} = \frac{1}{15.43} \times 437.5 = 28.35 \text{ gm}$$

$\therefore$ 1 ounce (Avoir) = 28.35 gr.

4. How many ml are in 1 fl. oz.

1 fl. oz = 480 m

16.23 m = 1 ml

$$1 \text{ m} = \frac{1}{16.23} \text{ ml}$$

$$480 \text{ m} = \frac{1}{16.23} \times 480 = 29.57 \text{ ml}$$

$\therefore$ 1 fl. oz = 29.57 ml.

5. Convert 3 drachm into mgs.

1 drachm = 60 gr

3 drachm = 60 × 3 = 180 gr

1 gr = 64.8 mg

180 gr = 64.8 × 180 = 11664 mg

$\therefore$ 3 drachm = 11664 mg.

6. Convert 550 mg into grains.

64.8 mg = 1 gr

$$1 \text{ mg} = \frac{1}{64.8} \text{ gr}$$

$$550 \text{ mg} = \frac{1}{64.8} \times 550 = 8.48 \text{ gr.}$$

7. Convert $\frac{1}{100}$ gr into metric weights.

$$1 \text{ gr} = 64.8 \text{ mg}$$

$$\frac{1}{100} \text{ gr} = 64.8 \times \frac{1}{100} = 0.648 \text{ mg.}$$

8. Convert $\frac{1}{6}$ gr into mgs.

$$1 \text{ gr} = 64.8 \text{ mg}$$

$$\frac{1}{6} \text{ gr} = 64.8 \times \frac{1}{6} = 10.8 \text{ mg.}$$

9. Convert 30 m into ml.

$$16.23 \text{ m} = 1 \text{ ml}$$

$$1 \text{ m} = \frac{1}{16.23} \text{ ml}$$

$$30 \text{ m} = \frac{1}{16.23} \times 30 = 1.848 \text{ ml.}$$

10. Convert 2 pt into ml.

$$1 \text{ pt} = 20 \text{ fl. oz}$$

$$2 \text{ pt} = 20 \times 2 = 40 \text{ fl. oz}$$

$$1 \text{ fl. oz} = 29.57 \text{ ml}$$

$$40 \text{ fl. oz} = 29.57 \times 40 = 1182.8 \text{ ml}$$

$$\therefore \quad 2 \text{ pt} = 1182.8 \text{ ml.}$$

Calculations based on Imperial systems

For preparing 1% w/v solns any of the following formulas which are identical in strength can be used :

	I	II	III	IV
Solid	1 gr	4.375 gr	35 gr	1 oz (Avoir)
Solvent to produce	110 m	1 fl. oz	8 fl. oz	100 fl. oz

Formula I should be used when the volume of the solution required is small and the strength of such solution is weak. Formula II, III & IV may be used according to the quantities of the solutions to be prepared.

While using formula I it is important to note that it is not permitted to weigh less than 1 gr of solid on the dispensing balance because of its low sensitivity. Hence, the volume prepared may be much more than the required volume. The excess volume so prepared may be rejected or preserved for further prescriptions to be dispensed.

1. *Rx*

Atropine sulphate ½%
Aqua q.s. ℨ ii

Calculations

1 gr of atropine sulphate dissolved in 110 m = 1% W/V soln
1 gr of atropine sulphate dissolved in 220 m = ½% W/V soln.

Dispense 120 m or 2 drachms out of the above soln and reject the remainder.

2. Prepare 1 oz of ⅛% solution of zinc sulphate in equal volumes of normal saline solution and adrenaline solution.

Calculations

Since two solvents, i.e., normal saline solution and adrenaline solution are used out of which adrenaline solution is costlier than normal saline solution therefore dissolve zinc sulphate at double strength in normal saline solutions.

1 gr of zinc sulphate dissolved in 110 m of normal saline solution = 1% W/V soln

1 gr of zinc sulphate dissolved in 440 m of normal saline solution = ¼% W/V soln

Take out 240 m of the above solution and mix it with 240 m of adrenaline solution. The resulting 480 m (1 oz) solution will be ⅛%.

3. Prepare 4 oz of 5% solution of a substance.

Calculations

35 gr dissolved in 8 fl. oz = 1% W/V soln

35×5 gr dissolved in 8 fl. oz = 5% W/V soln

$\frac{35 \times 5}{8}$ gr dissolved in one fl. oz = 5% W/V soln

$\frac{35 \times 5 \times 4}{8} = 87.5$ gr dissolved in 4 fl. oz = 5% W/V soln

Therefore, weigh 87.5 gr of the substance and dissolve in sufficient amount of water to produce 4 fl. oz. The resulting solution will be 5% solution.

4. Send 1 pint of a 1 in 500 solution of potassium permanganate.

Calculations

35 gr of potassium permanganate dissolved in 8 fl. oz = 1% W/V soln

$35 \times \frac{100}{500}$ gr of potassium permanganate dissolved in 8 fl. oz

$= \frac{1}{5}$ % W/V soln (1 in 500)

$\frac{35 \times 100}{500 \times 8}$ gr of potassium permanganate dissolved in one fl. oz

$= \frac{1}{5}$ % W/V soln

$\frac{35 \times 100 \times 20}{500 \times 8} = 17.5$ gr of potassium permanganate dissolved in 20 fl. oz

$= \frac{1}{5}$ % W/V soln

Therefore, weigh 17.5 gr of potassium permanganate and dissolve in sufficient amount of water to produce 1 pint. The resulting solution will be 1 in 500 solution.

5. How many tablets each containing 8.75 gr of mercuric chloride will be required to make one quart of 0.05% solution.

Calculations

35 gr dissolved in 8 fl. oz = 1% W/V soln

35×0.05 gr dissolved in 8 fl. oz = 0.05 % W/V soln

$\frac{35 \times 0.05}{8}$ gr dissolved in one fl oz = 0.05% W/V soln

$\frac{35 \times 0.05}{8} \times 40 = \frac{35 \times 5 \times 40}{8 \times 100} = 8.75$ gr dissolved in 40 fl. oz

= 0.05% W/V soln

8.75 gr of mercuric chloride contained in 1 tablet

1 gr of mercuric chloride contained in $\frac{1}{8.75}$ tablet

8.75 gr of mercuric chloride will be contained in $\frac{1}{8.75} \times 8.75$

= 1 tablet.

Therefore, each tablet of 8.75 gr of mercuric chloride will make one quart of 0.05% solution.

Solutions dispensed in concentrated form

6. Required 6 oz of a solution so that 2 teaspoonfuls diluted to a pint will make a 1 in 1000 solution.

This problem will be solved in two parts.

(a) Calculate the no. of grains required to make one pint of a 1 in 1000 solution.

(b) Every two teaspoonfuls of the concentrated solution must contain these number of grains. Therefore multiply these number of grains with the number of two teaspoonfuls contained in 6 oz.

(a) 35 gr dissolved in 8 fl. oz = 1 in 100 soln

$\frac{35 \times 100}{1000}$ gr dissolved in 8 fl. oz = 1 in 1000 soln

$\frac{35 \times 100}{1000 \times 8}$ gr dissolved in one fl. oz = 1 in 1000 soln

$\frac{35 \times 100 \times 20}{1000 \times 8} = 8.75$ gr dissolved in 20 fl. oz = 1 in 1000 soln.

Therefore, 8.75 gr of the drug must be contained in every 2 teaspoonfuls of the solution.

(b) 6 oz = $6 \times 8 = 48$ teaspoonfuls

2 teaspoonfuls contain 8.75 gr

1 teaspoonful contains = $\frac{8.75}{2}$ gr

48 teaspoonfuls must contain $\frac{8.75}{2} \times 48 = 210$ gr.

Therefore, dissolve 210 gr of the drug in water and dilute to 6 fl oz.

Sometimes concentrated solutions may be prescribed and the pharmacist is asked to label with directions to prepare weaker percentage solutions.

7. Send 4 oz of a 10% solution of potassium permanganate and label with directions for preparing a quart of a 1 in 400 solution.

Calculations

These types of problems are also calculated in two parts.

(a) Calculate the number of grains required to make 4 oz of a 10% solution.

(b) Calculate the quantity to be diluted to a quart to make a 1 in 400 solution.

(a) 35 gr dissolved 8 fl. oz = 1% W/V soln

35×10 gr dissolved in 8 fl. oz = 10% W/V soln

$\frac{35 \times 10}{8}$ gr dissolved in one fl. oz = 10% W/V soln

$\frac{35 \times 10 \times 4}{8} = 175$ gr dissolved in 4 fl. oz = 10% W/V soln.

Therefore, dissolve 175 gr in water and dilute it to 4 fl. oz.

(b) A 10% solution means 1 in $\frac{100}{10}$ = 1 in 10 soln.

That is, 10 oz of the solution contains 1 oz of the substance or, 10 oz of this solution diluted to 400 oz will produce 1 in 400 solution

or, $\frac{10 \times 40}{400}$ = 1 oz diluted to one quart will produce 1 in 400 solution.

Therefore, label with direction to dilute 1 oz or 2 tablespoonfuls to a quart.

Exercises (A)

Calculate the quantities required to prepare the following :

1. Atropine sulphate 1%. Send 4 drachms.
2. Acriflavine 0.1% in a mixture of equal volume of alcohol and water. Send 2 oz.
3. 8 oz of a 1 in 2000 solution.
4. 1 gallon of a 1 in 1000 solution.
5. 1 pint of a 0.01% solution.
6. 4 oz of a 0.625% solution.
7. 1 quart of a normal saline solution.
8. How many tablets each containing 8.75 gr of corrosive sublimate will be required to make 1 pint of a 0.4% solution.
9. 8 oz of a solution so that 1 tablespoonful to half a gallon makes 1 in 500 solution.
10. 8 oz so that 1 tablespoonful to half a gallon will make a 1 in 2000 solution.
11. 10 oz of a 2.5% solution and label with the directions for preparing a quart of 0.0625% solution.
12. 10 oz of 6% solution and label with the directions for preparing 30 oz of a 0.05% solution.
13. From 20% solution supplied prepare a quart of a 0.0625% solution.
14. From 8% solution supplied prepare 1 pint of a 1 in 1000 solution.

Calculations based on metric system

1. Calculate the formula for 40 gm coal tar and zinc ointment from the official formula given below :

Yellow soft paraffin	600 gm
Zinc oxide, finely sifted	300 gm
Strong coal tar solution	100 gm

Quantities required for 40 gm = $\frac{40}{1000}$ × official quantities.

2. Calculate the formula for 250 ml of oily lotion of calamine from the formula given below :

Calamine	50 gm
Wool fat	10 gm
Oleic acid	5 ml
Arachis oil	500 ml

Calcium hydroxide solution sufficient to produce 1000 ml

Quantities required for 250 ml = $\frac{250}{1000}$ × quantities given.

3. *Rx*

Hyoscine hydrobromide 0.6 mg

Make powders. Send such 10 powders.

Calculations

To get the required quantities for 10 powders, multiply the given quantity by 10.

4. *Rx*

Heavy magnesium carbonate	8.125 gm
Light magnesium carbonate	8.125 gm
Rhubarb, in powder	6.25 gm
Ginger, in powder	2.5 gm

Make powder. Send 100 gm.

Calculations

To get the required quantities for 100 gm, multiply the given quantities by 4.

Percentage Calculations

(i) *Weight in Volume (W/V) Solutions*

In this the solute is weighed and the solvent is measured. The general formula for 1% W/V solution is :

Solid	1 part by weight
Solvent to produce	100 parts by volume.

1 gm solute dissolved in sufficient amount of water to produce 100 ml or 10 mg in 1 ml of water makes 1% W/V solution.

Unless and until specially specified the solutions in pharmacy are supplied as W/V solutions.

(ii) *Weight in Weight (W/W) Solutions*

In this the solute and the solvent are taken by weight. The general formula for 1% W/W solution is :

Solid	1 part by weight
Solvent to produce	100 parts by weight.

Percentage solutions of solids in liquids are not made W/W unless specially requested.

(iii) *Volume by Volume (V/V) Solutions*

In this solute and the solvent are taken by volume. The general formula for 1% V/V solution is :

Solute	1 part by volume
Solvent to produce	100 parts by volume.

1 ml solute dissolved in sufficient amount of solvent to produce 100 ml.

5. Calculate the quantity of sodium chloride required to prepare 500 ml of a 2% solution.

   Calculations

   1 gm of sodium chloride dissolved in water to produce 100 ml
   = 1% W/V soln.

   1×2 gm of sodium chloride dissolved in water to produce 100 ml
   = 2% W/V soln.

   For 500 ml the quantity of sodium chloride required

   $$= \frac{1 \times 2 \times 500}{100} = 10 \text{ gm.}$$

   Therefore, dissolve 10 gm of sodium chloride in sufficient amount of water to produce 500 ml. The resulting solution will be 2% solution.

6. Calculate the quantity of sodium chloride required for preparing 200 ml of a 0.9% solution.

   Calculations

   1 gm of sodium chloride dissolved in water to produce 100 ml
   = 1% W/V soln.

   1×0.9 gm of sodium chloride dissolved in water to produce 100 ml
   = 0.9% W/V soln.

   For 200 ml the quantity of sodium chloride required

   $$= \frac{1 \times 0.9 \times 200}{100} = 1.8 \text{ gm.}$$

   Therefore, dissolve 1.8 gm of sodium chloride in sufficient amount of water to produce 200 ml. The resulting solution will be 0.9% solution.

7. Prepare 30 ml of 10% solution of methyl salicylate in alcohol.

   Calculations

   For 100 ml solution the quantity of methyl salicylate required
   = 10 ml

For 30 ml solution the quantity of methyl salicylate required

$$= \frac{10 \times 30}{100} = 3 \text{ ml.}$$

Therefore, mix 3 ml of methyl salicylate with sufficient alcohol to produce 30 ml. The resulting solution will be 10% solution.

8. Prepare 50 ml of 0.1% solution of acriflavine in a mixture of equal volume of alcohol and water.

Calculations

Alcohol is relatively expensive but water is inexpensive, therefore, prepare the acriflavine solution at double strength in water and then add alcohol.

Double the strength of 0.1% = 0.2%

1 gm of acriflavine dissolved in 100 ml of water = 1% W/V soln.

1×0.2 gm of acriflavine dissolved in 100 ml of water

= 0.2% W/V soln.

For 50 ml solution the quantity of acriflavine required

$$= \frac{1 \times 0.2 \times 50}{100} = 0.1 \text{ gm} = 100 \text{ mg.}$$

Therefore, dissolve 100 mg of acriflavine in 50 ml water. Out of this, measure 25 ml and mix it with 25 ml alcohol. The resulting solution will be 0.1% solution of acriflavine in a mixture of equal volume of alcohol and water.

9. Prepare 100 ml of a 1 in 4000 solution of potassium permanganate.

Calculations

$$1 \text{ in } 4000 = \frac{100}{4000} \text{ per cent} = 0.025\%$$

1 gm of potassium permanganate dissolved in 100 ml water

= 1% W/V soln.

1×0.025 gm of potassium permanganate dissolved in 100 ml water

= 0.025% W/V soln.

For 100 ml solution the quantity of potassium permanganate required

$$= \frac{1 \times 0.025 \times 100}{100} = 0.025 \text{ gm} = 25 \text{ mg.}$$

Therefore, dissolve 25 mg of potassium permanganate in sufficient water to produce 100 ml. The resulting solution will be 1 in 4000 solution.

10. Send 150 ml of 4% potassium permanganate solution and label with directions for preparing 500 ml of a 1 in 2500 solution.

Calculations

(a) 1 gm of potassium permanganate dissolved in 100 ml water = 1% W/V soln.

1×4 gm of potassium permanganate dissolved in 100 ml water = 4% W/V soln.

For 150 ml the quantity of potassium permanganate required

$$= \frac{1 \times 4 \times 150}{100} = 6 \text{ gm.}$$

Therefore, dissolve 6 gm of potassium permanganate in sufficient water to produce 150 ml solution.

(b) Strength of concentrated solution = 4%

Strength of dilute solution = 1 in 2500 = $\frac{100}{2500} = \frac{1}{25} = 0.04\%$

Degree of dilution = $\frac{4}{0.04}$ = 100 times.

Quantity of concentrated solution required = $\frac{500}{100}$ = 5 ml.

Therefore, dilute 5 ml of concentrated potassium permanganate soln upto 500 ml with water. The resulting solution will be 1 in 2500 solution.

11. From 1 in 400 solution of acriflavine, prepare 100 ml of 1 in 5000 solution.

Calculations

Strength of concentrated acriflavine soln provided

$$= 1 \text{ in } 400 = \frac{100}{400} = \frac{1}{4} = 0.25\%$$

Strength of dilute solution = 1 in 5000 = $\frac{100}{5000} = \frac{1}{50} = 0.02\%$

Degree of dilution = $\frac{0.25}{0.02} = \frac{25}{2}$ times.

Quantity of concentrated solution required = $\frac{100 \times 2}{25}$ = 8 ml.

Therefore, dilute 8 ml of concentrated solution of acriflavine upto 100 ml with water. The resulting solution will be 1 in 5000 solution.

Alcohol Dilutions

Dilute alcohols are made from 95% alcohol which contains 95 parts ethyl alcohol and 5 parts water. All other dilutions of alcohol are prepared by mixing the specified parts of alcohol and water.

On mixing alcohol with water, contraction in volume and rise in temperature occurs and mixture becomes turbid. The turbidity is caused by minute air bubbles evolved from the alcohol on dilution. Because air is less soluble in water than in alcohol, so on addition of water air is partly expelled from the solution. Since there will be contraction in volume and rise in temperature, consequently it is necessary to cool the mixture to about 20°C before adjusting to the final volume.

The general formula for calculating the amount of stronger alcohol required to make a weaker alcohol is as under :

Volume of stronger alcohol to be used

$$= \frac{\text{volume required} \times \text{percentage required}}{\text{percentage used}}$$

12. Prepare 600 ml of 60% alcohol from 95% alcohol.

Calculations

Volume of 95% alcohol to be used $= \dfrac{600 \times 60}{95} = 379$ ml.

Therefore, take 379 ml of 95% alcohol, dilute it upto 600 ml with water. The resulting dilution will contain 60% alcohol.

13. Prepare 500 ml of 40% alcohol from 95% alcohol.

Calculations

Volume of 95% alcohol to be used $= \dfrac{500 \times 40}{95} = 210$ ml.

Therefore, dilute 210 ml of 95% alcohol upto 500 ml with water. The resulting dilution will contain 40% alcohol.

Weight in Weight (W/W) Solutions

The general formula is as under :

Weight of stronger acid to be used

$$= \frac{\text{weight required} \times \text{percentage required}}{\text{percentage used}}$$

14. Send 200 ml of a solution of acetic acid containing 4% of real acetic acid. The strength of real acetic acid is 33%.

Calculations

Weight of stronger acid to be used $= \dfrac{200 \times 4}{33} = 24.2$ gm.

Therefore, weigh 24.2 gm of real acetic acid and dilute it upto 200 ml with water. The resulting solution will contain 4% acetic acid.

15. Send 200 ml of a solution of ammonia containing 4% by weight of ammonia. The strong solution of ammonia contains 32.5% of ammonia W/W.

Calculations

The weight of strong ammonia required = $\frac{200 \times 4}{32.5}$ = 24.615 gm.

Therefore, dilute 24.615 gm of strong solution of ammonia to 200 gm with water. The resulting solution will contain 4% ammonia.

Alligation Method

The calculations for exercises from 12 to 15 may be done by a method known as alligation method. This method is not recommended except as a method of checking because there are chances of errors in writing the figures.

16. Prepare 1000 gm of dilute acetic acid 4% from 33% real acetic acid.

Calculations

The weight of real acetic acid required = $\frac{1000 \times 4}{33}$ = 121.2 gm

The amount of water required = 1000 – 121.2 = 878.8 gm.

By alligation method

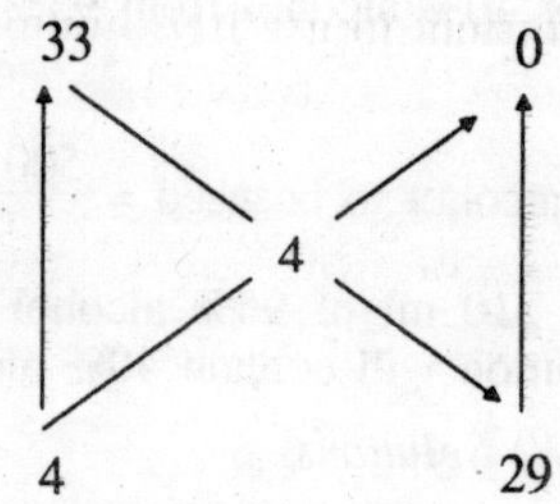

Subtract 0 (for water) from 4 = 4

Subtract 4 from 33 = 29

4 parts of real acetic acid and 29 parts of water will constitute 33 parts by weight of dilute acetic acid.

Therefore, the quantity of real acetic acid required

$$= \frac{1000 \times 4}{33} = 121.2 \text{ gm}$$

and the quantity of water required = $\frac{1000 \times 29}{33}$ = 878.8 gm.

17. Prepare 400 ml of 70% alcohol from 95% alcohol.

Calculations

Volume of 95% alcohol to be used = $\frac{400 \times 70}{95}$ = 294.74 ml

Volume of water to be used = 400 – 294.74 = 105.26 ml.

By alligation method

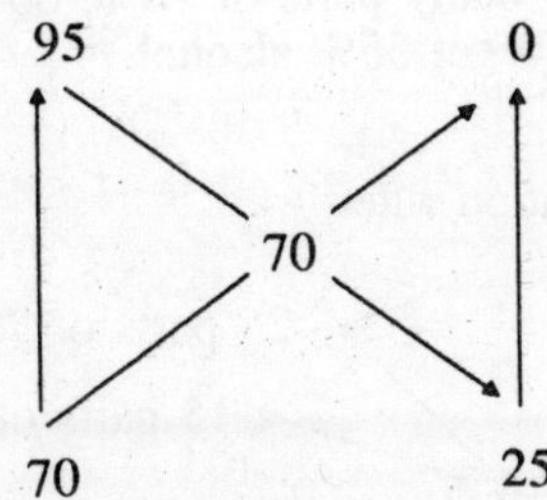

Subtract 0 (for water) from 70 = 70
Subtract 70 from 95 = 25
70 parts of 95% alcohol and 25 parts of water will constitute the required % alcohol.

$\therefore$ quantity of 95% alcohol required = $\frac{400 \times 70}{95}$ = 294.74 ml

and the quantity of water required = $\frac{400 \times 25}{95}$ = 105.26 ml.

18. Find out the quantity of 3% ointment which must be added to 100 gm of a 15% ointment to get 10% ointment.

Calculations

By applying alligation rule

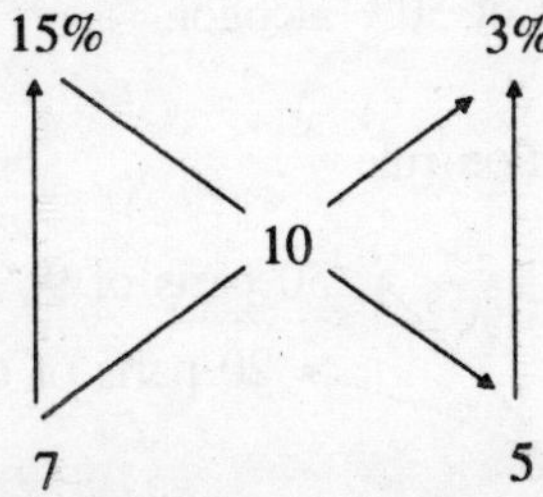

i.e., 7 parts of 15% ointment and 5 parts of 3% ointment must be mixed to get 10% ointment. The given strength of 100 gm ointment is 15%. So find out the relative proportion of 3% ointment required.

7 parts of 15% ointment require 5 parts of 3% ointment

1 part of 15% ointment requires $\frac{5}{7}$ parts of 3% ointment

100 parts of 15% ointment require $\frac{5}{7} \times 100$ parts of 3% ointment

$= \frac{500}{7}$ = 71.43 gm of 3% ointment.

Therefore, 71.43 gm of 3% ointment should be mixed with 100 gm of 15% ointment to get 10% ointment.

19. Find out that how many parts of 70%, 60%, 40% and 30% alcohol should be mixed to get 55% alcohol.

Calculations

By applying alligation rule

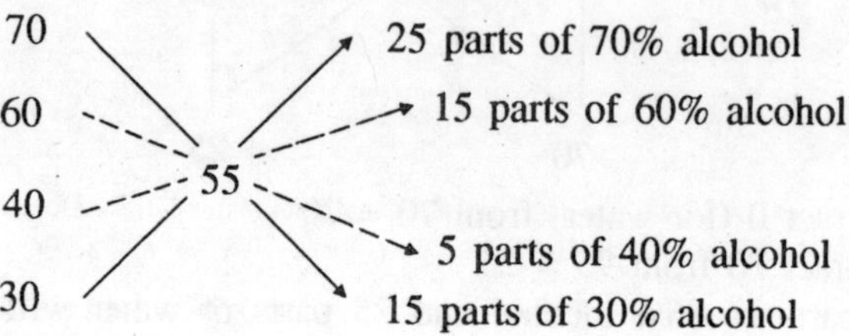

Therefore, when 25 parts of 70% alcohol, 15 parts of 60% alcohol, 5 parts of 40% alcohol and 15 parts of 30% alcohol are mixed together, the resulting solution will produce 55% alcohol.

Check :

$(25 \times 70) + (15 \times 60) + (5 \times 40) + (15 \times 30)$

$= 1750 + 900 + 200 + 450 = 3300$

$(25 + 15 + 5 + 15)\ 55 = 60 \times 55 = 3300.$

20. Find out the amount of each of 90%, 60%, 30% and water required to produce 500 ml of 50% alcohol.

Calculations

By applying alligation rule

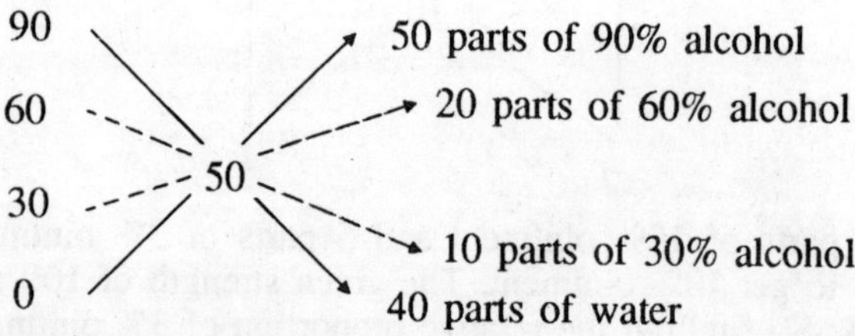

Therefore, when 50 parts of 90% alcohol, 20 parts of 60% alcohol, 10 parts of 30% alcohol and 40 parts of water are mixed together, the resulting solution will produce 50% alcohol.

Check :

$(50 \times 90) + (20 \times 60) + (10 \times 30) + (40 \times 0)$

$= 4500 + 1200 + 300 + 0 = 6000$

$(50 + 20 + 10 + 40)\ 50 = 120 \times 50 = 6000.$

Exercises (B)

1. Prepare 500 ml of 1 in 5000 solution of potassium permanganate.
2. Send 100 ml of 2% acriflavine solution.
3. Supply 500 ml of normal saline solution.
4. Prepare 300 ml of 45% alcohol from 90% alcohol.
5. Prepare 400 ml of 55% alcohol from 95% alcohol.
6. Send 200 ml of 60% alcohol from 95% alcohol.
7. Supply 500 ml of 20% alcohol from 95% alcohol.
8. From 90% alcohol provided supply 400 ml of 60% alcohol.
9. From 60% alcohol supplied prepare 2 litres of 45% alcohol.
10. Supply 250 ml of solution containing 15% of real acetic acid. The strength of official acetic acid is 33.
11. Prepare 120 ml of solution containing 20% of real acetic acid. The real acetic acid is 33% W/W.
12. Prepare 1000 gm of 6% acetic acid from 33% acetic acid.

Isotonic Solutions

All the ophthalmic and injectable solutions should be isotonic, e.g., ophthalmic solutions should be isotonic with lachrymal secretions (tears) to prevent irritation and pain, similarly, injectable solutions should be isotonic with blood plasma. Solutions having the same osmotic pressure are said to be isotonic. As compared to blood plasma if a solution has lower osmotic pressure it is said to be hypotonic but if it has higher osmotic pressure it is said to be hypertonic.

The solutions which are not isotonic with plasma may be harmful to use. On injecting the hypotonic solutions into blood stream, it may enter the red blood cells in an attempt to produce equilibrium, the cells swell rapidly until they burst leading to haemolysis. As this damage is irreversible, it may lead to serious danger to red blood cells.

When hypertonic solution is injected into the blood stream, the water comes out of the membrane of red blood cells in order to reach equilibrium. The cells shrink leading to crenulation which is only a temporary damage. When the osmotic pressure of two solutions becomes equal, the damaged cells will come to their original position. Hence hypertonic solutions may therefore be administered without permanent damage to the blood cells. They should be injected slowly to ensure rapid dilution into the blood stream and to minimise the crenulation of blood cells.

For the adjustment of tonicity of injectable solutions, substances like sodium chloride and dextrose, etc., are added. About 0.9% solution of sodium chloride is isotonic, 0.45% solution is hypotonic and 5% solution of sodium chloride is hypertonic with plasma.

Proof Spirit

For excise purposes, the strengths of alcoholic preparations are indicated by degrees "over proof" (O.P.) or "under proof" (U.P.). Proof spirit is legally defined as that mixture of alcohol and water which at 51°F weighs 12⁄13th of an equal volume of water. In India and Britain, this standard is equal to 57.1% V/V or 49.28% W/W of ethyl alcohol. Such a spirit has a sp. gr. of 0.91976 at 15.5°C. Whereas in USA 50% V/V of ethyl alcohol is considered to be 100 proof.

Any alcoholic solution which contains 57.1% V/V alcohol is a proof spirit and is said to be 100 proof. Any strength above proof strength is expressed as over proof (O.P.) and any strength below proof strength is expressed as under proof (U.P.). In India the rates of excise duty are charged in terms of rupees per litre of proof alcohol.

Any % V/V of alcohol can be converted into proof strength and vice versa by using the following method :

Multiply the % strength of alcohol by 1.753 and deduct 100 from the product. If the result is positive it is known as over proof and if the result is negative then it is known as under proof.

The figure 1.753 is obtained as follows :

57.1 volumes of ethyl alcohol = 100 volume of proof spirit

$$1 \text{ volume of ethyl alcohol} = \frac{100}{57.1} = 1.753 \text{ volumes of proof spirit}$$

Example 1. Find the strength of 90% V/V alcohol in terms of proof spirit.

Applying the formula

$$90 \text{ volumes of ethyl alcohol} = 90 \times 1.753 - 100 = 157.77 - 100$$
$$= +57.77 \text{ or } 57.77° \text{ O.P.}$$

Example 2. Calculate the real strength of 40° O.P. and 50° U.P.

Applying the formula

40 over proof means 100 + 40 = 140

$$\text{Alcohol strength} = \frac{140}{1.753} = 79.86\% \text{ V/V}$$

50 under proof means 100 – 50 = 50

$$\text{Alcohol strength} = \frac{50}{1.753} = 28.52\% \text{ V/V}$$

Check if strength is 79.86% V/V and 28.52% V/V value of proof will be

(i) $79.86 \times 1.753 - 100 = 139.99 - 100 = +39.99$ or 40° O.P.

(ii) $28.52 \times 1.753 - 100 = 49.99 - 100 = -50.01$ or 50° U.P.

Example 3. A sample of brandy is 30 under proof. Calculate its alcoholic strength V/V.

30 under proof means 30 – 100 = 70

$$\text{Alcoholic strength} = \frac{70}{1.753} = 39.93 \text{ or } 40\% \text{ V/V.}$$

Example 4. How many proof gallons are contained in 4 gallons of 70% V/V alcohol.

Applying the formula

$$\begin{aligned} \text{Value of proof} &= \% \text{ strength of alcohol} \times 1.753 - 100 \\ &= 70 \times 1.753 - 100 = 122.71 - 100 \\ &= +22.71 \quad \text{or } 22.71° \text{ O.P.} \end{aligned}$$

That means

$$\begin{aligned} 100 \text{ gallons of } 70\% \text{ V/V alcohol} &= 100 + 22.71 \\ &= 122.71 \text{ gallons of proof spirit} \end{aligned}$$

$$1 \text{ gallon of } 70\% \text{ V/V alcohol} = \frac{122.71}{100} \text{ gallons of proof spirit}$$

$$\begin{aligned} 4 \text{ gallons of } 70\% \text{ V/V alcohol} &= \frac{122.71}{100} \times 4 \text{ gallons of proof spirit} \\ &= 4.90 \text{ gallons of proof spirit} \end{aligned}$$

Therefore, 4 gallons of 70% V/V alcohol are equivalent to 4.90 gallons of proof spirit.

Exercises (C)

1. Convert the following strength of alcohol into proof spirit :
   (i) 70.74% V/V (ii) 50.16% V/V
   (iii) 25.78% V/V (iv) 79.87% V/V
   (v) 47.31% V/V
2. Convert the following degree of proof spirit into % V/V strength of alcohol :
   (i) 44.6° O.P. (ii) 18.4° O.P.
   (iii) 35.3° O.P. (iv) 75.0° U.P.
   (v) 54.8° U.P.
3. How many proof gallons are represented by 50 wine gallons of 90% V/V alcohol.

Answers

(A)

1. 3 gr of atropine sulphate to be dissolved in sufficient water to produce 330 m.
2. Take 1 gr acriflavine and dissolve it in sufficient water to produce

550 m. Out of this measure out 480 m and mix it with 480 m alcohol. Produce the final volume to 2 oz because there will be little contraction in volume which occurs when alcohol is diluted with water.

3. 1.750.
4. 70.0 gr.
5. 0.875 gr.
6. 10.9375 gr.
7. 157.5 gr.
8. 4 tablets.
9. 70 gr, 1120 gr.
10. 17.5 gr, 280 gr.
11. 109.375 gr, two tablespoonful to be diluted to a quart.
12. 262.5 gr, two teaspoonful to be diluted to 30 oz.
13. ⅛ oz or 60 minims. 14. ¼ oz or 120 minims.

(B)

1. Dissolve 100 mg potassium permanganate in sufficient water to produce 500 ml solution.
2. Dissolve 2 gm acriflavine in sufficient water to produce 100 ml solution.
3. Dissolve 4.5 gm sodium chloride in sufficient water to produce 500 ml solution.
4. 150 ml.
5. 231.578 ml.
6. 126.315 ml.
7. 105.263 ml.
8. 266.666 ml.
9. 1.5 lit.
10. 113.636 gm.
11. 72.72 gm.
12. 181.818 gm.

(C)

1. (i) 24° O.P. (ii) 12.07° U.P. (iii) 54.81° U.P. (iv) 40° O.P. (v) 17.07° U.P.
2. (i) 82.48% V/V (ii) 67.54% V/V (iii) 77.18% V/V (iv) 14.26% V/V (v) 25.78% V/V.
3. 78.88 proof gallons.

Revision Questions

I. Very short answer type questions

Answer the following questions in brief

(i) What is prescription?

(ii) Name various parts of a prescription?

(iii) Why Latin language is used in prescription writing?

(iv) What is the importance of writing the word RJ in prescription writing?

II. Fill in the blanks

(a) Prescription is a ...... order by the prescriber to the ....
(b) The Latin word used for writing the directions to the patient is ....
(c) The signature of the prescriber must be written ....
(d) While collecting and weighing the materials for compounding a prescription the label on every stock bottle must be read at least ...... times.
(e) The prescription must be received and checked by the ......

III. Short answer type questions

1. What is the importance of date in prescription writing?
2. Discuss the importance of name, age and address of the patient in the prescription.
3. Describe in brief the importance of age in the prescription.
4. Give an example of a representative prescription.

IV. Long answer type questions

1. What is 'prescription'? Describe various parts of a prescription.
2. Define the term 'prescription'. Describe different parts and significance of each part of an ethical prescription.
3. Explain the term 'prescription'. Describe the procedure that low a prescription is to be handled by a pharmacist.
4. What is the importance of label to be fixed on a pharmaceutical formulation? Discuss what information is required to be written on label.
5. Translate the following Latin terms into English :
   (i) Ad libitum.
   (ii) Agita
   (iii) Alternis horis
   (iv) a.c.
   (v) Applicandus
   (vi) b.i.d.
   (vii) Cataplasma
   (viii) Cum parte aequale
   (ix) Coch-parvum
   (x) Congius
   (xi) Dol. urg.
   (xii) E. lacte
   (xiii) Ex. Modo prescripto
   (xiv) Guttae
   (xv) Hora somni
   (xvi) Inter cibos

(xvii) Levis
(xviii) m
(xix) Modo dicto
(xx) Nocte maneque
(xxi) o.d.
(xxii) Omni quardanta hora
(xxiii) Nebula
(xxiv) Omni mane
(xxv) p.a.a.
(xxvi) p.p.a.
(xxvii) Post cibos
(xxviii) Pro dosi
(xxix) Pro-re neta
(xxx) q.s.
(xxxi) Secudum artum
(xxxii) Si opus sit (s.o.s.)
(xxxiii) Solve
(xxxiv) Statim
(xxxv) Tales
(xxxvi) Ter quotidie
(xxxvii) Tussi urgente
(xxxviii) Quinque
(xxxix) Decem
(xxxx) Duodecim.

Answers

5. (a) Written, Pharmacist; (b) Sig; (c) By his own hand with ink; (d) Three; (e) Pharmacist

2

Pharmaceutical Incompatibilities

A pharmaceutical incompatibility may be defined as the result of prescribing or mixing the substances which are antagonistic in nature and an undesirable product is formed which may affect the safety, purpose or appearance of the preparation. These incompatibilities are of three general types, i.e., physical, chemical and therapeutic.

Physical incompatibilities are those when two or more than two substances are combined together, a physical change takes place and an unacceptable product is formed. Since these changes which take place are usually visible therefore they can be easily corrected by applying the pharmaceutical skill to obtain an acceptable preparation.

Chemical incompatibilities are those in which a chemical reaction takes place between the ingredients and a new undesirable compound is formed. These types of incompatibilities are little difficult to correct and in some cases it may be necessary to eliminate or substitute one of the reacting substances, dispense them in separate containers, change them to non-reactive form or to pack and store in suitable containers. In such cases the physician should be consulted and informed.

THERAPEUTIC INCOMPATIBILITY

Therapeutic incompatibility may be the result of prescribing certain drugs to the patient with the intention to produce a specific degree of action but the nature or the intensity of the action produced is different from that intended by the prescriber. It may be due to the administration of (i) overdose or improper dose of a single drug; (ii) wrong dose or dosage form; (iii) contraindicated drugs; (iv) synergistic and antagonistic drugs.

Rx

Codeine phosphate 0.6 gm

Make powders. Send such 10 powders.

Type : Therapeutic incompatibility.

In the present prescription an overdose of codeine phosphate has been prescribed. Therefore the prescription must be referred back to the prescriber.

Rx

Tetracycline hydrochloride 250 mg

Make capsules. Send such 10 capsules.
Label : Take one capsule every six hours with milk.
Type : Therapeutic incompatibility.

In this prescription the direction is wrong. Tetracycline is, inactivated by calcium which is present in milk. Therefore tetracycline capsules should not be taken with milk. Hence refer back the prescription to the prescriber for the directions to be changed.

*R*x

Amphetamine sulphate	20 mg
Ephedrine sulphate	100 mg
Simple syrup	up to 100 ml

Make a mixture.
Type : Therapeutic incompatibility.

In the present prescription two drugs i.e. amphetamine sulphate and ephedrine sulphate have been prescribed, both of which are sympathomimetic in action with additive effect. So there is need to reduce the dose of each drug. Hence the prescription should be referred back to the prescriber.

*R*x

Acetophenatidin	150 mg
Acetyl salicylic acid	200 mg
Caffeine	40 mg

Make capsules. Send such 10 capsules.
Type : Therapeutic incompatibility (Intentional)

In this prescription both the drugs i.e. Acetophenatidin and Acetyl salicylic acid are analgesic. Acetophenatidin is CNS depressant (this side effect is undesirable) whereas caffeine is CNS stimulant, which neutralises the side effect of acetophenatidin. This is an intentional incompatibility, so dispense the prescription as such.

Although the physician is responsible for the prescribed medications but the pharmacist must be aware of the possibility of errors and whenever he finds some error in the prescription, he must consult the prescriber for the correct dispensing of prescription. This will save the prescriber, the pharmacist and the patient from serious consequences.

Incompatibilities of physical and chemical type may be either instantaneous or delayed. In the first case visual changes like effervescence, liquefaction or precipitation may take place. In the delayed incompatibilities the reaction or changes take place at a later stage, e.g., crystallization, cracking of emulsions or colour change, etc.

Now a days the prescriptions are generally written for the official and proprietary preparations which are prepared by the pharmaceutical industries and are available in pharmaceutical prepackaged form. Rarely the prescriptions are compounded by the pharmacist but even then the pharmacist must be conversant with the incompatibilities which take place in compounding the pharmaceutical preparations. By applying the pharmaceutical, chemical and pharmacological background he must decide the most suitable line of action to get the desired product.

PHYSICAL INCOMPATIBILITY

Physical incompatibility is usually due to immiscibility, insolubility, precipitate formation or liquefaction of solid materials. This usually causes non-uniform, unsightly or unpalatable mixtures. Sometimes it becomes very difficult to measure an accurate dose from non-uniform products. Usually these types of difficulties can be easily overcome by applying the pharmaceutical skill to present the product with the best possible appearance and to ensure uniform doses of medication. Generally physical incompatibilities may be corrected by one or more of the following method, i.e., order of mixing, alteration of solvents, change in the form of ingredients, alteration of volume, emulsification, addition of suspending agent; addition, substitution or omission of therapeutically inactive substances to facilitate the compounding of the prescription.

Examples of Physical Incompatibilities and Their Methods of Correction

1. Oils and water are immiscible with each other. They can be made miscible by emulsification, e.g., castor oil emulsion, olive oil emulsion, liquid paraffin emulsion, etc.

Rx

Olive oil	30 ml
Water	up to 120 ml

Make an emulsion.
Type : Physical incompatibility.

In this prescription olive oil (a fixed oil) is immiscible with water. To make them miscible, an emulsifying agent will have to be incorporated.

2. In liquid preparations containing indiffusible solids such as prepared chalk, acetyl salicylic acid, succinyl sulphathiazole, sulphadimidine, phenacetin, zinc oxide and calamine, etc., a suspending agent will have to be incorporated so as to increase the thickness of the preparation and to maintain uniform distribution of the substances for sufficiently long time after shaking the bottle thus facilitating uniform measurement of each dose.

Rx

Phenacetin	3 gm
caffeine	1 gm
Orange syrup	12 ml
Water	up to 90 ml

Make a mixture.

In this prescription phenacetin is an indiffusible substance, so to make it diffusible a suspending agent, either compound tragacanth powder or tragacanth mucilage, will have to be used.

3. Certain powders like sulphur, antibiotics and certain corticosteroids are insoluble in water and are difficult to wet with water. Some wetting agents like saponins or polysorbates may be used to distribute these powders in water.
4. Resins are insoluble in water, therefore when a resinous tincture is added to water the resin forms indiffusible clots which can be prevented either by slowly adding the undiluted tincture with vigorous stirring to the diluted suspension, or by adding some suitable thickening agent.
5. Oils dissolved in alcohol separate out on the addition of water.
6. High concentrations of electrolytes cause cracking of soap emulsions by salting out the emulsifying agent.
7. Addition of a common solvent in an emulsion which may dissolve the oily phase, the aqueous phase and the emulsifying agent lead to the formation of one phase system, e.g., addition of alcohol in turpentine liniment.
8. Certain low melting point solids, when mixed together liquefy due to the formation of eutectic mixtures. Substances when any two of them are mixed together liquefy or form a soft mass include camphor, menthol, thymol, phenol, chloral hydrate, sodium salicylate, acetyl salicylic acid and phenazone.

These types of substances create problem when they are to be dispensed in powder form. For this purpose they can either be triturated together to form liquid and mixed with an absorbent like light kaolin or light magnesium carbonate to give a free flowing product or each ingredient is powdered separately and mixed with an absorbent and then combined together lightly and filled in suitable containers.

Rx

Menthol	5 gm
Camphor	5 gm
Ammonium chloride	30 gm
Light magnesium carbonate	60 gm

Make an insufflation.

Type : Physical incompatibility.

In the above prescription, menthol, camphor and ammonium chloride are liquefiable substances. When any two of them are combined together they liquefy and form a eutectic mixture. Therefore to dispense them in powders light magnesium carbonate is added which acts as an absorbent.

CHEMICAL INCOMPATIBILITY

Chemical incompatibility may be result of chemical interactions between the ingredients of a prescription and a harmful or even dangerous product may be formed. Therefore precautions should be taken either to prevent the formation of harmful product or to correct them. In such cases the prescriber must be informed.

Generally chemical incompatibilities result from oxidation reduction, acid-base, hydrolysis or combination reactions. These reactions may be noticed by precipitation, effervescence, decomposition, colour change or by explosion and usually occur immediately when the prescription ingredients are mixed and thus these types of incompatibilities are called immediate incompatibilities. They should be dispensed only after correction. Sometimes the reactions proceed at a very slow rate and no appreciable visible change occurs which may develop on standing. Such types of incompatibilities are known as delayed incompatibilities. These types of incompatibilities may or may not result in loss of therapeutic activities.

Types of Chemical Incompatibilities

The chemical incompatibilities fall into two groups :

(a) Tolerated

In tolerated incompatibilities, where practicable the reaction is minimised by applying some suitable order of mixing or mixing the solutions in dilute forms but no alteration is made in the active ingredients of the preparation.

(b) Adjusted

In adjusted incompatibilities the reaction is prevented by addition or substitution of one of the reacting substances with another of equal therapeutic value but does not affect the medicinal action of the preparation (e.g., substitution of caffeine citrate with caffeine in sodium salicylate and caffeine citrate mixtures).

The incompatibility may be (i) intentional when the prescriber knowingly prescribes the incompatible drugs or (ii) it may be un-intentional when the prescriber prescribes the drugs without knowing that there is incompatibility in the prescribed drugs.

General Methods for Precipitate Yielding Combinations

Generally, it is noticed that reaction between strong solutions proceed at a faster rate and the precipitates formed are thick and do not diffuse readily whereas the reaction between the dilute solutions proceed at a slow rate and the precipitates formed are light and diffuse readily in the solution. Hence the reacting substances should be diluted to the maximum extent before mixing them. The precipitates so formed may be diffusible or indiffusible. The methods adopted for dispensing such prescriptions in which diffusible or indiffusible precipitates are formed will be described under the heading method A and method B.

Method A

This method is used when diffusible precipitates are formed and in those cases where the amount of precipitates formed is very small.

Divide the vehicle into two equal portions. Dissolve one of the reacting substances in one portion and the other in the other portion. Mix the two portions by slowly adding one portion to the other with rapid stirring.

Method B

This method is used when the indiffusible precipitates are formed and they form an appreciable portion of the mixture.

Divide the vehicle into two equal portions. Dissolve one of the reacting substances in one portion. Place the other portion of the vehicle in a mortar, to this incorporate a suitable amount of compound tragacanth powder (10 grains per ounce or 2 gm per 100 ml of the finished product) with constant trituration until a smooth mucilage is produced, then add and dissolve the other reacting substances. Mix the two portions by slowly adding one portion to the other with rapid stirring.

Whether method A or method B has been used in dispensing the prescription, it is very important to fix a "Shake the bottle." label to the container and ensure that the patient strictly follows and realises the importance of these directions.

Methods of Correcting Chemical Incompatibilities

1. Alkaloidal Salts with Alkaline Substances

Most alkaloidal salts are soluble in water but alkaloidal bases are practically insoluble in water and are freely soluble in organic solvents.

When an alkaline substance like aromatic spirit of ammonia, solution of ammonia, ammonium bicarbonate, sodium bicarbonate, potassium bicarbonate, borax, etc., is added to an alkaloidal salt solution the free alkaloid may be precipitated. However they are not always precipitated, because all alkaloids are slightly soluble in water and other added substances as for example :

(a) Strychnine

Tincture nux vomica is generally used as a source of strychnine in mixtures required to stimulate the appetite. The amount of strychnine present is 0.125 gm per 100 ml of tincture nux vomica and the solubility of strychnine is about 1 in 7000, i.e., 100 ml of water will dissolve

$$\frac{1 \times 100}{7000} = 0.143 \text{ gm of strychnine.}$$

Hence the amount of strychnine present in 10 ml of tincture nux vomica will be easily dissolved in 100 ml of water and will not be precipitated in alkaline solutions. Further, tinctures contain certain amount of alcohol due to which the precipitation is further prevented. Moreover the solubility of strychnine is much more in alcohol (i.e., 1 in 150) than in water. Therefore it follows that in mixtures containing sufficient amount of alcohol strychnine will not be precipitated even when more than 10 ml of tincture per 100 ml is present in the prescription.

Rx

Strychnine hydrochloride solution	6 ml
Aromatic spirit of ammonia	4 ml
Water	120 ml

Make a mixture.

Type : Chemical incompatibility (incompatibility of alkaloidal salts with alkaline substances).

Strychnine hydrochloride is an alkaloidal salt and aromatic spirit of ammonia is an alkaline substance. When they react together the precipitates of strychnine are formed because the quantity of strychnine hydrochloride prescribed is much more than its solubility, moreover the amount of alcohol present in aromatic spirit of ammonia is also negligible, hence strychnine gets precipitated. The precipitates so formed are diffusible in nature. Therefore follow method A for precipitate-yielding combinations.

(b) Morphine

The solubility of morphine is 12 minim per ounce. Therefore, preparations containing less than 12 minim per ounce of morphine will not be precipitated with alkaline substances. Further, morphine is more soluble in alcohol (i.e., 1 in 100) than in water. Therefore, in mixtures containing sufficient alcohol morphine will not be precipitated even if more than 12 minim per ounce is prescribed along with alkaline substances.

(c) Solanaceous Alkaloids

Tincture belladonna, tincture hyoscyamus and tincture stramonium containing solanaceous alkaloids are generally prescribed in mixtures, and the contents of these alkaloids in the prescribed amount is very low therefore are not precipitated in the alkaline solutions. Moreover presence of alcohol in tinctures further decreases precipitation.

(d) Ipecacuanha Alkaloids

Tincture ipecacuanha which contains emetine is mainly used in cough mixtures which may also contain alkaline substances like sodium bicarbonate or ammonium bicarbonate but emetine is not precipitated because the quality of tincture prescribed is very low and presence of alcohol further prevents precipitation.

(e) Codeine

Codeine is soluble in 120 parts of water or 2 parts of alcohol, because of its appreciable solubility in water the codeine is not precipitated from dilute solutions of its salts when mixed with alkaline substances.

(f) Caffeine

Caffeine is soluble in 80 parts of water or 40 parts of alcohol. It will not be precipitated in the doses prescribed in the prescriptions.

(g) Cocaine

Cocaine is slightly soluble in water (i.e., 1 in 1300) but fairly soluble in alcohol (1 in 10). Cocaine hydrochloride is generally used in eye drops, nasal sprays and throat sprays. In the presence of alkaline substances cocaine is precipitated therefore such formulations should not be dispensed. Cocaine eye drops must be dispensed in alkali-free containers.

(h) Quinine

Quinine is slightly soluble in water but very soluble in alcohol. Quinine is generally precipitated in mixtures when a normal dose of soluble quinine salt is prescribed with an alkaline substance so it should not be dispensed. However powders containing quinine and acetyl salicylic acid can be dispensed and used safely but they should not be kept and stored for a long time because darkening, and decomposition may take place, in which case they should be discarded.

2. Alkaloidal Salts with Soluble Iodides

Potassium iodide is generally prescribed as an expectorant in some of the cough mixtures also containing alkaloids but the quantity of alkaloids present (e.g., emetine from ipecacuanha tincture) is usually so low that the precipitation of hydriodide is unlikely to take place.

Strychnine when combined with soluble iodides forms a very insoluble hydriodide, the precipitates of which are diffusible hence follow method A for precipitate-yielding combinations.

3. Alkaloidal Salts with Tannins

When an alkaloidal salt is combined with a drug containing tannins, the alkaloids form tannates which are insoluble in water and the precipitates so formed are usually diffusible in nature therefore follow method A for precipitate-yielding combinations.

Since most alkaloids form insoluble tannates therefore this fact is frequently used in the treatment of alkaloidal poisoning in which case a strong solution of tannic acid or strong tea is administered which will precipitate the alkaloid and render it less harmful.

4. Alkaloidal Salts with Salicylates

Generally quinine compounds are prescribed with salicylates in the treatment of malaria. When quinine is combined with salicylates it forms indiffusible precipitates of quinine salicylate therefore follow method B for precipitate-yielding combinations.

Rx

Quinine hydrochloride	130 mg
Sodium salicylate	4 gm
Water	up to 90 ml

Make a mixture.

Type : Chemical incompatibility (incompatibility of alkaloidal salts with salicylates).

Quinine hydrochloride reacts with sodium salicylate to form the precipitates of quinine salicylate which are indiffusible in nature. Therefore follow method B for precipitate-yielding combinations.

Rx

Sodium salicylate	1.0	gm
Caffeine citrate	0.650	gm
Water	up to 30.0	ml

Make draught.

Type : Chemical (adjusted) incompatibility.

Caffeine citrate is a mixture of equal weights of caffeine and citric acid. The citric acid present reacts with sodium salicylate to liberate salicylic acid which gets precipitated. But if caffeine is used instead of caffeine citrate, it forms a soluble complex with sodium salicylate.

Therefore substitute half as much caffeine as that of caffeine citrate and a clear mixture will be obtained.

5. Soluble Salicylates with Alkali Bicarbonates

When sodium salicylate is administered orally, it reacts with hydrochloric acid present in the stomach, liberating salicylic acid which is precipitated and leads to irritation of the gastric mucosa and pain in the stomach. Hence when sodium salicylate is prescribed it is usually given along with double the quantity of sodium bicarbonate as that of sodium salicylate, thereby partially neutralising the gastric secretion and thus minimising the formation and precipitation of salicylic acid.

When sodium salicylate is dispensed in the solution form, especially along with an alkaline substance like sodium bicarbonate the mixture absorbs oxygen from the atmosphere and becomes reddish brown in colour. This change does not significantly affect the therapeutic effectiveness of the medicament but may lead to confusion in the mind of the patient that the medicament has spoiled and he may not like to take it, therefore to avoid this confusion a colouring agent like liquid extract of liquorice or extract of burnt sugar may be added to darken the above mentioned mixture. If this is not done, the patient should be warned about the colour change. The colour change can also be retarded by adding an antioxidant such as sodium metabisulphite 0.1 percent but this should be added with the permission of the prescriber.

Rx

Sodium salicylate	1.0	gm
Sodium bicarbonate	1.0	gm
Sodium metabisulphite	0.01	gm
Chloroform water	up to 15.0	ml

Fiat mistura.

Type : Simple mixture.

When sodium salicylate comes in contact with hydrochloric acid present in stomach, salicylic acid is formed which gets precipitated and leads to irritation in the stomach. Hence when sodium salicylate is prescribed it is usually prescribed with sodium bicarbonate which will temporarily neutralise the gastric secretion and thus minimise the formation of salicylic acid.

Sodium salicylate in solution form, specially when it is alkaline in nature, absorbs oxygen and solution becomes brownish black. Though the therapeutic value is not changed but it may lead to confusion in the mind of the patient that the mixture has spoiled and he may not like to use the mixture. Therefore to prevent the air oxidation, sodium metabisulphite is used as an antioxidant which will considerably retard the change in colour.

6. Soluble Salicylates and Benzoates with Acids

Most of the acids and acid syrups like syrup lemon B.P.C. which contain citric acid decompose sodium salicylate and sodium benzoate with the formation and precipitation of salicylic acid and benzoic acid respectively. The precipitates so formed are indiffusible in nature therefore follow method B for precipitate-yielding combinations. Otherwise syrup lemon which contains citric acid can be replaced (with the permission of the prescriber) without altering the therapeutic action of the preparation, with simple syrup and tincture lemon.

Rx

Sodium salicylate	5 gm
Syrup of lemon	20 ml
Water	up to 75 ml

Make a mixture.

Type : Chemical (adjusted) incompatibility.

Syrup of lemon contains citric acid. When it reacts with sodium salicylate, salicylic acid is formed which gets precipitated; the precipitates of which are indiffusible in nature.

Syrup of lemon is prescribed as a flavouring agent which can be replaced without altering the therapeutic action of the preparation. Therefore replace syrup of lemon with 19 ml of simple syrup and 1.2 ml of tincture of lemon.

7. Soluble Salicylates with Ferric Salts

Ferric salts react with sodium salicylate with the formation of precipitates of ferric salicylate which are indiffusible in nature. Therefore follow method B for precipitate-yielding combinations. In the presence of sodium bicarbonate the precipitates of ferric salicylate remain soluble therefore a clear mixture is obtained.

Rx

Ferric chloride solution	2 ml
Sodium salicylate	4 gm
Water	up to 90 ml

Make a mixture.

Type : Chemical incompatibility (incompatibility of salicylates with ferric salts).

Ferric chloride reacts with sodium salicylate to form ferric salicylate, the precipitates of which are indiffusible in nature. Hence follow method B for precipitate-yielding combinations.

8. Potassium Chlorate with Oxidisable Substances

When potassium chlorate is prescribed with an oxidisable substances like tannic acid, sugar, sulphur or any other readily oxidisable substance and heated or triturated together, there are chances of explosion. Therefore these dry substances should not be triturated together. They should be powdered separately in a dry and clean mortar and then mixed together lightly with a bone spatula on a paper or ointment slab without any friction.

9. Incompatibilities Causing Evolution of a Gas

When carbonates or bicarbonates are dispensed in the presence of an acid or acidic drug, they react together with the evolution of carbon dioxide. If the reaction is not allowed to complete and the mixture is transferred immediately to the bottle and corked there are chances of explosion with bursting of the bottle.

To prevent explosion, mix the ingredients in an open vessel and allow the reaction to complete until effervescence ceases. When whole of the carbon dioxide goes out, transfer the mixture to the bottle and cork. In some cases where the reaction proceeds slowly hot vehicle should be used to hasten the reaction.

(a) Borax with Sodium Bicarbonate and Glycerin

When borax and glycerin are mixed together, hydrolysis of borax takes place with the formation of sodium metaborate and boric acid. The boric acid so formed reacts with glycerin to form monobasic glyceryl boric acid. Boric acid itself is a weak acid therefore will not react with carbonates or bicarbonates whereas monobasic glyceryl boric acid formed is sufficiently strong to react with bicarbonates to liberate carbon dioxide.

$$\underset{\text{(Borax)}}{Na_2B_4O_7} + 3H_2O \rightarrow \underset{\text{(Sodium metaborate)}}{Na_2B_2O_4} + \underset{\text{(Boric acid)}}{2H_3BO_3}$$

$$\underset{\text{(Boric acid)}}{3H_3BO_3} + \underset{\text{(Glycerin)}}{2C_3H_5(OH)_3} \rightarrow \underset{\text{(Monobasic glyceryl boric acid)}}{(C_3H_5)_2(HBO_3)_3} + 6H_2O$$

When these three substances are to be compounded they should be mixed in an open vessel and mixture should not be transferred to the bottle until effervescence ceases. Hot water should be used as vehicle to hasten the reaction.

Rx

Sodium bicarbonate	1.5	gm
Borax	1.5	gm
Phenol	0.75	gm
Glycerin	25.00	gm
Water	up to 100.00	ml

Make a spray solution.

Type : Chemical incompatibility (incompatibility of evolution of carbon dioxide).

When sodium bicarbonate, borax and glycerin are mixed together in the presence of water, a reaction takes place with the evolution of carbon dioxide. If the mixture is dispensed as such, there are chances of bursting the bottle. Therefore mix these substances in an open vessel until evolution of carbon dioxide ceases. Incorporate phenol and transfer the mixture to the bottle.

(b) Bismuth Subnitrate and Sodium Bicarbonate

In the presence of water bismuth subnitrate reacts with sodium bicarbonate liberating carbon dioxide. This reaction proceeds slowly at ordinary temperature, hence the reaction should be accelerated by using hot water and mixture should not be transferred to the bottle until the effervescence ceases.

$$\underset{\text{(Bismuth subnitrate)}}{2BiONO_3} + 2NaHCO_3 \rightarrow \underset{\text{(Bismuth subcarbonate)}}{(BiO)_2CO_3} + 2NaNO_3 + CO_2 + H_2O$$

(c) Sodium Bicarbonate with Soluble Calcium or Magnesium Salts

When sodium bicarbonate is combined with soluble calcium or magnesium salts, double decomposition reaction takes place with the formation of corresponding insoluble carbonate and carbon dioxide. The precipitates of carbonates formed are diffusible in nature, so follow method A for precipitate-yielding combinations.

$$MgSO_4 + 2NaHCO_3 \rightarrow Mg(HCO_3)_2 + Na_2SO_4$$

$$\underset{\text{(Magnesium bicarbonate)}}{4Mg(HCO_3)_2} \rightarrow 3MgCO_3 + \underset{\text{(Magnesium hydroxide)}}{Mg(OH)_2} + 5CO_3 + 3H_2O$$

At ordinary temperature the reaction proceeds slowly, hence it should be accelerated by using the vehicle hot and mixture should not be bottled until effervescence ceases.

10. Liquid Extract of Liquorice in Acid Media

Liquid extract of liquorice has its flavouring properties due to the presence of glycyrrhizin, which is a sweet substance consisting of calcium and potassium salts of glycyrrhizinic acid. When liquid extract of liquorice is used as a flavouring agent in acid mixtures, the acid reacts with glycyrrhizin forming glycyrrhizinic acid which is precipitated and a sticky black sediment is formed which is difficult to diffuse. With the precipitation of glycyrrhizinic acid the flavouring property of the liquid extract is destroyed therefore it should not be used as flavouring agent in acid mixtures and should be used only in neutral or alkaline solutions. If prescribed in acid mixtures, the prescription should be referred back to the prescriber for substitution of a suitable flavouring agent.

11. Soluble Barbiturates with Ammonium Bromide

When soluble barbitone or soluble phenobarbitone is combined with ammonium bromide in the presence of water, a reaction takes place with the formation of barbitone which is insoluble in water therefore precipitated and precipitates so formed are indiffusible in nature, hence follow method B for precipitate-yielding combinations.

When soluble phenobarbitone is prescribed with ammonium bromide, it can be assumed that the prescriber intends the patient to receive a clear mixture, which can be produced by replacing chemically equivalent amount of ammonium bromide with sodium bromide or potassium bromide. Since the qualitative action of these bromides is the same, i.e., they produce sedative action therefore ammonium bromide can be replaced with sodium bromide or potassium bromide to get a clear mixture.

Rx

Phenobarbitone sodium	650 mg
Ammonium bromide	8 gm
Water	up to 120 ml

Make a mixture.

Type : Chemical incompatibility (incompatibility of soluble barbiturates with ammonium bromide).

In this prescription phenobarbitone sodium reacts with ammonium bromide with the formation of indiffusible precipitates of phenobarbitone. But if ammonium bromide is replaced with an equivalent amount of either sodium bromide or potassium bromide, a clear mixture is obtained. The pharmacological action of these three bromides is the same, but the intensity of action depends on the amount of bromide radicals used.

$$NH_4Br = NaBr$$
$$98 = 103$$
(mol. wt. of NH_4Br = 98, mol. wt. of NaBr = 103)

For 98 gm of NH_4Br the amount of NaBr required = 103 gm

For 1 gm of NH_4Br the amount of NaBr required = $\frac{103}{98}$ gm

For 8 gm of NH_4Br the amount of NaBr required = $\frac{103}{98} \times 8$ gm = 8.4 gm.

Therefore replace 8 gm of ammonium bromide with 8.4 gm of sodium bromide and prepare the mixture as such. The resulting mixture will be a clear mixture.

Revision Questions

I. Very short answer type questions

Answer the following questions in brief

1. What is incompatibility?
2. Define the term 'physical incompatibility'?
3. Define the term 'chemical incompatibility'?
4. What do you understand from the term 'therapeutic incompatibility'?
5. Mention different types of incompatibility?
6. What is tolerated incompatibility?
7. What is adjusted incompatibility?
8. Name different kinds of precipitates formed during chemical incompatibility?

II. Short answer type questions

1. Fill in the blanks :
   (a) Incompatibility is of ...... types.
   (b) Method A for precipitate yielding combinations is used for ...... precipitates.
   (c) Method B for precipitate yielding combinations is used for ...... precipitates.
   (d) Oil and water are ...... with each other.
   (e) When two or more than two low melting point solids are mixed to gather, they liquefy. Such substances are known as ...... :
   (f) Capsules of tetracycline hydrochloride are never advised to be taken with ...... because tetracycline gets inactivated due to presence of ...... in milk.
   (g) Alkaloidal salts when dispensed with ...... substances, the free alkaloid may be precipitated.
   (h) Incompatibility between phenobarbitone sodium and ammonium bromide is removed by ...... ammonium bromide with ......
   (i) Liquid extract of liquorice has its flavouring properties due to the presence of ......
2. Write short notes on :
   (a) Physical incompatibility
   (b) Chemical incompatibility
   (c) Therapeutic incompatibility
   (d) Eutectic substances.
3. Differentiate between :
   (a) Physical, chemical and therapeutic incompatibility.
   (b) Tolerated and adjusted incompatibility.
   (c) Intentional and unintentional incompatibility.

4. How will you dispense following combination of drugs in mixtures? Give reasons thereof :
   (a) Strychnine hydrochloride with an alkaline substance.
   (b) Sodium salicylate and caffeine citrate.
   (c) Sodium salicylate and sodium bicarbonate.
   (d) Sodium salicylate with syrup of lemon.
   (e) Borax, glycerin and sodium bicarbonate.
   (f) Alkali bicarbonates with soluble calcium or magnesium salts.
   (g) Iodides with ferric salts in the presence of alkali salts
   (h) Glycyrrhiza liquid extract with acidic substances
   (i) Phenobarbitone sodium and ammonium bromide.

III. Long answer type questions

1. Define 'incompatibility' Explain various types of incompatibilities giving suitable examples.
2. What is incompatibility? Discuss the reasons why physical and therapeutic incompatibility occurs. Describe the method to correct such incompatibilities.
3. How will you dispense the following prescriptions? Explain the incompatibility involved and suggest methods to correct them :

(a) R_x

Castor oil	30 ml
Water	up to 120 ml

Fiat emulsio. Mitte 60 ml.

(b) R_x

Menthol	10 gm
Camphor	10 gm
Ammonium chloride	60 gm
Light magnesium carbonate	120 gm

Fiat insufflatio. Mitte 40 gm.

(c) R_x

Sodium salicylate	1.0 gm
Caffeine citrate	0.65 gm
Water	up to 30.0 ml

Make draught.

(d) R_x

Sodium bicarbonate	1.5 gm
Borax	1.5 gm
Phenol	0.75 gm

Glycerin	25.0 gm
Water	up to 100.0 ml

Make a spray solution.

(e) R_x

Phenobarbitone sodium	650 mg
Ammonium bromide	8 gm
Water	up to 120 ml

Make a mixture. Send 60 ml.

(f) R_x

Tetracycline hydrochloride	250 mg

Fiat capsula. Mitte tales decem.
Label : One capsule to be taken every six hours with milk.

4. What is pharmaceutical incompatibility? Name various types of incompatibilities and explain chemical incompatibility in detail.

Answers

II. 1.

(a) Three
(b) Diffusible
(c) Indiffusible
(d) Immiscible
(e) Eutectic substances.
(f) Milk, calcium
(g) Alkaline
(h) Replacing, Sodium or Potassium bromide
(i) Glycyrrhizin.

3

Posology

The word posology is derived from the Greek words 'posos', meaning how much and 'logos', meaning science. That means it is a branch of medical science which deals with doses or quantity of drugs which can be administered to produce the required pharmacological actions.

The dose of a drug may be defined as the quantity of drug which is "enough but not, too much," the idea is to produce the drug's optimum therapeutic effect in a particular patient with the lowest possible dose. The pharmacopoeias and textbooks usually give a minimum and maximum dose for each drug. Minimum dose is necessary to produce a desired therapeutic effect but maximum dose is the largest quantity which can be given safely to an individual without producing harmful effects. Beyond the maximum dose certain toxic effects and undesirable effects may be produced.

The dose of a drug cannot be fixed rigidly because there are so many factors which influence the doses, e.g., age, condition of the patient, severity of the disease, natural tolerance, acquired tolerance, idiosyncrasy, route of administration, degree of absorption and rate of elimination. The doses listed below are not binding upon the prescriber, considering the above mentioned factors he can change the doses accordingly.

The doses mentioned in the table represent the average maximum quantities of drugs which can be administered to an adult orally within 24 hours; when other routes of administration are followed the relevant appropriate dose is mentioned. If the doses are to be administered in divided doses, the frequencies of administration are stated.

The doses given here are for general guidance. It is the responsibility of the prescriber regarding the amount of drug prescribed or the frequency at which the drug is administered. But before dispensing any medication it is the duty of the pharmacist to satisfy himself that overdose has not been prescribed. In case of doubt he should consult the prescriber and to confirm the doses of individual medicaments he can consult the extra pharmacopoeia.

DOSES PROPORTIONATE TO AGE

Calculation of Child Dose

The dose for a child from adult dose can be calculated by any one of the following formulas :

(A) According to Age

1. Young's Rule

$$\text{Child's dose} = \frac{\text{age in years}}{\text{age in years} + 12} \times \text{adult dose.}$$

For example, if the adult dose is 60 mg and the age of the child is 4 years, the dose for the child will be

$$\frac{4}{4+12} \times 60 = \frac{4}{16} \times 60 = \frac{1}{4} \times 60 = 15 \text{ mg}$$

2. Dilling's Rule

$$\text{Child's dose} = \frac{\text{age in years}}{20} \times \text{adult dose.}$$

For example, if the adult dose is 60 mg and the age of the child is 6 years, the dose for the child will be

$$\frac{6}{20} \times 60 = \frac{3}{10} \times 60 = 18 \text{ mg.}$$

Because of quicker and easy calculations, Dilling's rule is considered better.

3. Clark's Formula (according to body weight)

$$\text{Child's dose} = \frac{\text{child's weight (kg)}}{70} \times \text{adult dose.}$$

For example, if the adult dose is 60 mg and the weight of the child is 14 kg, the dose for the child will be

$$\frac{14}{70} \times 60 = 12 \text{ mg.}$$

DOSES PROPORTIONATE TO SURFACE AREA

The calculation of child's dose according to surface area is more appropriate rather than the methods based on age. This method is more complicated than the methods based on age but tables have been provided by which dose for a child can be calculated. This methods is based on the following formula :

$$\frac{\text{Surface area of child} \times 100}{\text{Surface area of adult}} = \text{Percentage of adult dose.}$$

Table

Age	*Percentage of adult dose*
One month	10
2 months	15
4 months	20
1 year	25
3 years	35
5 years	40
10 years	60
12 years	75
16 years	90

FACTORS AFFECTING DOSE AND ACTION OF DRUGS

Various factors which influence the dose and action of a drug in an individual are as follows :

1. Age

In determining the dose of a drug the age of an individual is of great significance specially in the young or very old persons. Children and old persons need lesser amount of drug than the standard adult dose because they are unable to inactivate or excrete drugs to that extent as adults but at the same time children can tolerate relatively large doses of digitalis and belladonna on the basis of their body weights as compared with adults. Newborn infants are abnormally sensitive to certain drugs because of the immature state of their hepatic and renal function by which drugs are normally inactivated and eliminated from the body.

2. Body Weight

Generally recommended adult doses are based on a "normal" body weight of 70 kg. But such a dose will be too less for a muscular person weighing 100 kg and too large for a weak person weighing about 50 kg. The calculation of doses for children on the basis of body weight is considered more dependable than that based strictly on age. The doses calculated according to body weight are expressed as mg/kg body weight.

3. Sex

Generally females require lesser dose than males because of their lesser weight and also due to the reason that they are more responsive to the effects of certain drugs than males. Drugs should be given very carefully during menstruation, pregnancy and lactation. Strong purgatives should be avoided during menstruation, whereas drugs which stimulate contraction of uterus should be avoided in pregnant ladies which may lead to abortion or miscarriage. Drugs like alcohol, anaesthetic gases, barbiturates, narcotic and non-narcotic analgesics, etc., which are readily transported from mother to the foetal circulation should be avoided. These drugs produce adverse effects to the foetus sometimes resulting in death of the foetus in the uterus. During lactation, drugs such as antihistaminics, morphine and tetracyclines which are excreted in milk should be given very cautiously to the mothers who are breast-feeding the babies.

4. Route of Administration

The dose of a given drug may vary according to the dosage form and route of administration used. Drugs administered intravenously enter the blood stream directly hence require lesser dose than the subcutaneous dose which in turn is smaller than the oral dose.

5. Time of Administration

Time of administration of drugs is very important. Drugs are rapidly absorbed from the empty stomach, hence an amount of drug that is effective when taken before a meal may be ineffective if administered during or after meals. On the other hand irritating drugs are better tolerated if administered after meals which will dilute the drug's concentration and reduce the gastric irritation, e.g., iron, arsenic, cod-liver oil, etc., should always be given on a full stomach.

6. Presence of Disease

Drugs are more effective in diseased conditions than normal body conditions. During fever one can tolerate high doses of antipyretics than in a nonfebrile condition. Similarly during hepatic or renal disturbances, the drugs which are metabolised in the liver or excreted through the kidneys may prove fatal.

7. Environmental Factors

Alcohol is better tolerated in cold environments than in summer. Dose of a sedative required to produce sleep during day time is much more than the dose required to produce sleep during night.

8. Emotional Factors

Females are more emotional and responsive to drugs therefore require less dose of drugs. The faith inspired by the doctor on the mind of a patient is an important factor in medication. Nervous patients require smaller doses of drugs as compared to normal patients.

9. Accumulation

When a drug is repeatedly administered for a long time, depending on its nature, it may unexpectedly accumulate in the body to produce sudden toxic symptoms. The drugs which produce such symptoms of poisoning are called cumulative drugs. The cumulative effects are usually produced by slow excretion, defective degradation or unexpectedly rapid absorption of drugs. Therefore drugs like digitalis, emetine, bromides, heavy metals should be carefully administered but cumulative effect is desirable in drugs like chloroquin and phenobarbitone which are used in cases of malaria and epilepsy respectively.

10. Synergism

When two or more drugs are used in the combined form their action is either increased or decreased depending on the drugs used in combination. When the potency or duration of action is increased, the phenomenon is called synergism. This synergism is of two types : (a) addition and (b) potentiation.

(a) Addition

When the total effect of two drugs is just equal to the sum of their individual effects, it is known as addition.

(b) Potentiation

When the combined effect of two drugs administered is greater than the sum of their individual effects, it is known as potentiation, e.g., combination of ephedrine and adrenaline acts as a better bronchodialator.

Synergism is very useful where desired therapeutic result needed is difficult to obtain with a single drug especially if single drug produces side effects. By this action dose of individual drugs can be lowered.

11. Antagonism

When the action of one drug is opposed by the other drug, the phenomenon is known as antagonism. The total combined effect is less than the algebraic total effect of the two drugs, e.g., milk of magnesia is given in acid poisoning. Here one drug is acidic and another is alkaline. They react with each other or in other words it may be said that the effect of one drug is antagonised by the other drug. Similarly if adrenaline and acetylcholine are given together they neutralise the effect of each other because adrenaline is vasoconstrictor whereas acetylcholine is vasodilator.

12. Habituation and Addiction

(a) Habituation

When repeated use of a drug or agent leads to production of emotional or psychological dependence rather than compulsion the condition is known as habituation, e.g., use of tea, coffee, tobacco, chewing of betel nut, tranquilizers, etc. When such agents are withdrawn the individual can carry on his routine work. Here there is no physical dependence, hence it can be easily tackled.

(b) Addiction

It is a state of psychic and physical drug dependence. Continuous use of alcohol, opium, cocaine, heroin, morphine, pethidine, LSD leads to addiction and turns the person to a wreck who becomes liability to society. The addicts are deeply attached to the drug and become slave of it, therefore craves for it at all times and tries to procure it by any means, fair or foul. If he is unable to get the drug, he develops withdrawal symptoms which may be serious enough to produce death. So the drugs which lead to addiction must be prescribed very cautiously.

13. Idiosyncrasy

All persons do not respond alike to the same drug due to varied individual susceptibility, some may produce abnormal reaction to a drug. When an abnormal or unusual reaction is produced by a drug it is known as idiosyncrasy, e.g., few mg of aspirin may produce gastric haemorrhage and small doses of quinine may produce ringing in the ear.

14. Hypersensitivity

Hypersensitivity is an allergic reaction to a drug and is different from either the expected pharmacological response or toxic reaction to the drug. This is due to frequent or indiscriminate use of drugs like antibiotics, vitamins and especially proteinous substances. Once a person is sensitised, a minute dose of the drug will produce allergic reactions. It is of two types (i) immediate type which is serious and requires prompt injection of adrenaline otherwise death may occur (ii) delayed type in which urticaria, skin rashes or contact dermatitis may occur.

15. Tolerance

When a drug administered in an ordinary dose fails to produce the normal therapeutic effect and requires large dose of the drug to produce the normal effect. The unusual resistance thus produced is known as tolerance, e.g., smokers can tolerate nicotine, alcoholics can tolerate large doses of alcohol, rabbits can tolerate large doses of atropine due to quick destruction of the drug by enzyme atropine estrase present in their blood.

Tachyphylaxis

It is also known as acute tolerance. It is observed in certain drugs that when they are administered repeatedly at very short intervals the cell receptors get blocked up and pharmacological response to that particular drug is decreased. By increasing the dose this decreased response cannot be reversed. But if the administration of the drug is stopped for a long time and administered again after being discontinued then the initial effect of the drug can be reobserved. This condition is known as tachyphylaxis. Drugs like ephedrine, amphetamine, cocaine, and nitrites behave in this way.

Doses of Different Drugs, their Route of Administration and Uses

Name of drug	*Maximum doses*	*Route of administration*	*Uses*
Adrenaline acid tartrate	0.4 to 1 mg	By s/c injection as single dose.	Sympathomimetic.
Adrenaline injection	0.2 to 0.5 ml	By s/c injection as single dose.	Sympathomimetic.
Aluminium hydroxide gel	7.5 to 15 ml	Oral.	Antacid.
Dried aluminium hydroxide gel	0.5 to 1 gm	Oral.	Antacid.
Aminophylline	100 to 300 mg	Oral.	Bronchodialator.
	250 to 500 mg	By slow 1/v injection.	
Amphetamine sulphate	5 to 20 mg	Oral, daily in divided doses.	Central nervous system stimulant.
Ampicillin	1 to 6 gm	Oral, daily in divided doses.	Antibiotic.
Amylobarbitone	100 to 200 mg	Oral.	Hypnotic.
Amylobarbitone sodium	400 mg	Oral, daily in divided doses.	Sedative.
Aneurine hydrochloride (Vit. B_1)	5 mg	Oral, daily prophylactic dose.	Vitamin B_1 deficiency.
	100 mg	Oral, daily therapeutic dose.	Vitamin B_1 deficiency.
	100 mg	By s/c or 1/m injection.	Vitamin B_1 deficiency.
Antazoline hydrochloride	100 to 300 mg	Oral, daily in divided doses.	Antihistaminic.
Apomorphine hydrochloride	2 to 8 mg	By s/c or 1/m injection.	As an emetic.
Ascorbic acid (Vit. C)	25 to 75 mg	Oral, prophylactic dose.	For preventing scurvy.
	250 mg	Oral, therapeutic dose.	For treating scurvy.
Aspirin (Acetyl salicylic acid)	0.3 to 1 gm	Oral.	Analgesic and antipyretic.
	4 to 8 gm	Oral, daily in divided doses.	In the treatment of acute rheumatism.
Atrophine sulphate	0.25 to 2 mg	Oral, daily in single or divided doses.	Parasympatholytic.
	0.25 to 2 mg	By s/c, 1/m or 1/v injection.	Parasympatholytic.
B.C.G. vaccine	0.1 ml	By intracutaneous injection as prophylactic dose.	Active immunisation against tuberculosis.

(*Contd.*)

Name of drug	*Maximum doses*	*Route of administration*	*Uses*
Barbitone sodium	300 to 600 mg	Oral.	As hypnotic.
	900 mg	Oral, daily in divided doses.	As sedative.
Belladonna dry extract	15 to 60 mg	Oral.	Antispasmodic.
Belladonna tincture	0.5 to 2 ml	Oral.	Antispasmodic.
Bemegride	1 gm	50 mg repeated at an interval of ten minutes by 1/v injection according to the need of the patient.	In the treatment of barbiturate poisoning.
Benzylpenicillin	0.5 to 3 gm	Oral, daily in divided doses.	Antibiotic.
	0.3 to 6 gm	By 1/m or 1/v injection daily in divided doses.	Antibiotic.
Butobarbitone	100 to 200 mg	Oral.	Hypnotic.
Caffeine	100 to 300 mg	Oral.	Central nervous system stimulant.
Caffeine citrate	100 to 300 mg	Oral.	Central nervous system stimulant.
Calciferol	20 mcg	Oral.	In the prevention of rickets.
	0.125 to 1.25 mg	Oral.	In the treatment of rickets and osteomalacia.
Calcium carbonate	1 to 5 gm	Oral.	Antacid.
Calcium gluconate	1 to 5 gm	Oral.	In the treatment of calcium deficiency.
	1 to 2 gm	By 1/m or 1/v injection.	
Calcium lactate	1 to 5 gm	Oral.	In the treatment of calcium deficiency.
Castor oil	5 to 20 ml	Oral.	Cathartic purgative.
Chloral hydrate	0.3 to 2 gm	Oral.	Hypnotic.
Chloramphenicol	1.5 to 3 gm	Oral, daily in divided doses.	Antibiotic.

Contd.

Name of drug	*Maximum doses*	*Route of administration*	*Uses*
Chlordiazepoxide	10 to 100 mg	Oral, daily in divided doses.	Tranquilizer.
Chloroform spirit	0.25 to 2 ml	Oral.	Flavour and preservative.
Chloroquin phosphate	500 mg	Oral, weekly	In suppression of malaria.
	0.5 to 1.5 gm	Oral, daily.	In the treatment of malaria.
	200 to 300 mg (base)	By 1/m or 1/v injection.	In the treatment of malaria.
	0.5 to 1 gm	Oral, daily in divided doses.	In the treatment of hepatic amoebiasis.
Chlorothiazide	0.5 to 2 gm	Oral.	Diuretic.
Chlorpheniramine maleate	4 to 16 mg	Oral, daily in divided doses.	Antihistaminic.
	5 to 20 mg	By 1/m injection as a single dose.	
Chlorpromazine hydrochloride	75 to 800 mg	Oral, daily in divided doses.	In psychiatric states.
	25 to 50 mg	Oral and by 1/m injection.	As an antiemetic.
Chlortetracycline hydrochloride	1 to 3 gm	Oral, daily in divided doses.	Antibiotic.
Codeine phosphate	10 to 60 mg	Oral.	In cough and diarrhoea; also acts as weak analgesic.
Cod-liver oil	10 ml	Oral.	In the prevention of rickets.
Cortisone acetate	50 to 400 mg	Oral and by 1/m injection daily in divided doses.	Corticosteroid.
Cyanocobalamin (Vit. B_{12})	1 mg	Initial dose by 1/m injection repeated ten times at intervals of two or three days.	In the treatment of vitamin B_{12} deficiency and in the treatment of megaloblastic anaemia.
	250 mcg	Maintenance dose by 1/m injection every four weeks until the blood count is normal.	In the treatment of vitamin B_{12} deficiency and in the treatment of megaloblastic anaemia.

(Contd.)

Name of drug	*Maximum doses*	*Route of administration*	*Uses*
Dexamethasone	10 mg	Oral, daily in divided doses.	Corticosteroid.
Diazepam	5 to 30 mg	Oral, daily in divided doses.	Tranquilizer.
	5 to 10 mg	By 1/m or slow 1/v injection.	
Digoxin	1.5 mg	Initial dose, in single or divided doses, for rapid digitalisation.	In the treatment of congestive heart failure.
	50 mcg	Maintenance dose, daily.	
Di-iodohydroxy-quinoline	1 to 2.0 gm	Oral, daily in divided doses.	In the treatment of amoebiasis.
Emetine hydrochloride	30 to 60 mg	By s/c or 1/m injection daily.	In the treatment of amoebiasis.
Ephedrine hydrochloride	15 to 60 mg	Oral.	In the treatment of asthma.
Ergometrine maleate	0.5 to 1 mg	Oral and by 1/m injection.	Uterine stimulant.
Ergotamine tartrate	1 to 2 mg	Oral.	In the treatment of migraine.
	250 to 500 mcg	By s/c or 1/m injection.	
Erythromycin	1 to 4 gm	Oral, daily in divided doses.	Antibiotic.
Erythromycin estolate	≡ 1 to 4 gm base	Oral, daily in divided doses for not more than 10 days.	Antibiotic.
Ferric ammonium citrate	1 to 6 gm	Oral, daily in divided doses.	In the prevention and treatment of iron deficiency anaemia.
Ferrous sulphate	300 mg	Oral, daily prophylactic dose.	In the prevention and treatment of iron deficiency anaemia.
	900 mg	Oral, in divided doses, daily therapeutic dose.	In the treatment of iron deficiency anaemia.
Folic acid	5 to 20 mg	Oral, daily.	In the treatment of megaloblastic anaemia.

(Contd.)

Name of drug	*Maximum doses*	*Route of administration*	*Uses*
	200 to 500 mcg	Oral, daily.	In prophylaxis of megaloblastic anaemia of pregnancy.
Frusemide	40 to 120 mg	Oral.	Diuretic.
Gentamycin sulphate	80,000 to 240,000 units	By 1/m injection daily, in divided doses.	Antibiotic.
Griseofulvin	0.5 to 1 gm	Oral, daily in divided doses.	Antifungal-antibiotic.
Halibut liver oil	0.2 to 0.5 ml	Oral.	Source of vitamin A.
Heparin	10,000 to 15,000 units	By 1/v or 1/m injection.	Anticoagulant.
Hydrocortisone acetate	5 to 50 mg	By intra-articular injection.	Corticosteroid.
Hyoscine hydrobromide	300 to 600 mcg	Oral and by s/c injection.	Central nervous system depressant and also used in motion sickness.
Hyoscyamus tincture	2 to 5 ml	Oral.	Central nervous system depressant and also used in motion sickness.
Ipecacuanha liquid extract	0.1 ml	Oral.	Expectorant and emetic.
Ipecacuanha tincture	1 ml	Oral.	Expectorant and emetic.
Isoniazid	300 to 600 mg	Oral, daily in divided doses.	Used in tuberculosis along with streptomycin.
Light kaolin	15 to 75 gm	Oral.	Antidiarrhoeal; antacid.
Liquid extract of liquorice	2 to 5 ml	Oral.	Expectorant.
Light and heavy magnesium carbonate	250 to 500 mg	Oral.	As an antacid.
	2 to 5 gm	Oral.	As a laxative.
Light magnesium oxide	250 to 500 mg	Oral.	As an antacid.
	2 to 5 gm	Oral.	As a laxative.

(Contd.)

Name of drug	*Maximum doses*	*Route of administration*	*Uses*
Liquid paraffin	10 to 30 ml	Oral	As a laxative.
Magnesium hydroxide mixture	5 to 10 ml	Oral.	As an antacid.
	25 to 50 ml	Oral.	As a laxative.
Magnesium sulphate	15 gm	Oral.	Purgative.
Magnesium trisilicate	0.5 to 2 gm	Oral.	As an antacid.
Male fern extract	3 to 6 ml	Oral.	In thread-worm infestation.
Meprobamate	0.4 to 1.2 gm	Oral, daily in divided doses.	Sedative.
Methyldopa	≡ 0.5 to 3 gm anhydrous methyldopa	Oral, daily in divided doses.	In the treatment of hypertension.
Morphine hydrochloride	10 to 20 mg	Oral.	Narcotic analgesic.
Morphine sulphate	10 to 20 mg	Oral, by s/c or 1/v injection.	Narcotic analgesic.
Nalorphine hydrobromide	5 to 10 mg	Initial dose by 1/v injection; repeated in accordance with patient's needs to a total dose not exceeding 40 mg.	Antidote for morphine poisoning.
Neomycin sulphate	1.4 to 4.2 mega units	Daily, in divided doses.	As an intestinal antiseptic.
Nicotinamide	15 to 30 mg	Oral, prophylactic.	A component of vitamin B complex.
	50 to 250 mg	Oral, daily therapeutic dose.	
Nicotinic acid	15 to 30 mg	Oral, prophylactic dose.	A component of vitamin B complex.
	50 to 250 mg	Oral, daily therapeutic dose.	
Nikethamide	0.5 to 2 gm	By 1/v injection.	Respiratory stimulant.
Noscapine	15 to 30 mg	Oral.	Cough suppressant.
Nux vomica liquid extract	0.05 to 0.2 ml	Oral.	Bitter tonic.
Nux vomica tincture	0.5 to 2 ml	Oral.	Bitter tonic.
Nystatin	1 to 2 mega units	Oral, daily in divided doses.	Antifungal antibiotic.

(*Contd.*)

Name of drug	*Maximum doses*	*Route of administration*	*Uses*
Oxyphenbutazone	200 to 400 mg	Oral, daily in divided doses.	Analgesic and anti-inflammatory.
Oxytetracycline hydrochloride	1 to 3 gm	Oral, daily in divided doses.	Antibiotic.
Paracetamol	0.5 to 1 gm	Oral.	Analgesic, antipyretic.
	up to 4 gm	Oral, daily in divided doses.	
Paraldehyde	5 to 10 ml	Oral and by 1/m injection.	Hypnotic, sedative, anti-convulsant.
	15 to 30 ml	By rectal injection.	As a basal anaesthetic.
Pentobarbitone sodium	100 to 200 mg	Oral.	Hypnotic.
Peppermint oil	0.05 to 0.2 ml	Oral.	Carminative and flavouring agent.
Pethidine hydrochloride	50 to 100 mg	Oral and by s/c and 1/m injection.	Narcotic analgesic.
	50 mg	By 1/v injection.	
Phenacetin	300 to 600 mg	Oral.	Analgesic and antipyretic.
Phenobarbitone	up to 350 mg	Oral, in divided doses.	Hypnotic, anti-convulsant.
Phenobarbitone sodium	up to 350 mg	Oral, in divided doses.	Hypnotic, anti-convulsant.
Phenolphthalein	50 to 300 mg	Oral.	Laxative.
Phenoxymethyl-penicillin	0.5 to 1.5 gm	Oral, daily in divided doses.	Antibiotic.
Phenylbutazone	200 to 400 mg	Oral, daily in divided doses.	Analgesic and anti-inflammatory.
Phthalylsulphathiazole	5 to 10 gm	Oral, daily in divided doses.	Antibacterial agent used in large intestine.
Piperazine citrate	1 to 2 gm	Oral, daily in divided doses.	In the treatment of thread-worm infestation.
Piperazine phosphate	4.5 gm	Oral, single dose.	In the treatment of round-worm infestation.

(*Contd.*)

Name of drug	*Maximum doses*	*Route of administration*	*Uses*
Potassium bromide	1 to 6 gm	Oral, daily in divided doses.	Sedative.
Potassium iodide	250 to 500 mg	Oral.	As an expectorant.
	150 mg	Oral, daily in divided doses.	In the preoperative treatment of thyrotoxicosis.
Prednisolone	5 to 60 mg	Oral, daily in divided doses.	Corticosteroid.
Prednisone	5 to 60 mg	Oral, daily in divided doses.	Corticosteroid.
Primaquin phosphate	≡ 15 mg base	Oral, daily for 14 days.	In the cure of malaria.
Procaine penicillin	300 to 900 mg	Daily by 1/m injection.	Antibiotic.
Progesterone	20 to 60 mg	Daily by 1/m injection.	Progestational steroid.
Pseudoephedrine hydrochloride	60 to 180 mg	Oral, daily in divided doses.	Used for the relief of nasal congestion.
Pyridoxine hydrochloride (Vit. B_6)	100 to 300 mg	Oral, daily in divided doses.	A component of vitamin B complex.
Quinine hydrochloride	300 to 600 mg	Oral, daily.	In suppression of malaria.
Quinine sulphate	1.2 to 2 gm	Oral, daily in divided doses.	In the treatment of malaria.
Reserpine	1 to 5 mg	Oral, daily in divided doses.	In psychiatric states.
	100 to 500 mcg	Oral, daily.	In the treatment of hypertension.
Riboflavine (Vit. B_2)	1 to 4 mg	Oral, prophylactic dose.	A component of vitamin B complex.
	5 to 10 mg	Oral, daily therapeutic dose.	
Smallpox vaccine	0.02 ml	Prophylactic dose by scarification or pressure inoculation.	In prevention of smallpox.
Sodium bicarbonate	1 to 5 gm	Oral.	As an antacid.
Sodium bromide	1 to 6 gm	Oral, daily in divided doses.	Sedative.
Sodium citrate	up to 10 gm	Oral, daily in divided doses.	Systemic alkalinising substance.

(Contd.)

Name of drug	*Maximum doses*	*Route of administration*	*Uses*
Sodium iodide	250 to 500 mg	Oral.	As an expectorant.
	150 mg	Oral, daily in divided doses.	In the preoperative treatment of thyrotoxicosis.
Sodium salicylate	5 to 10 gm	Oral, daily in divided doses.	In the treatment of acute rheumatism.
Streptomycin sulphate	≡ 500 mg base	Oral, every eight hours.	As an intestinal antiseptic.
	≡ 1 gm base	By 1/m injection daily or at longer intervals.	
Sulphadiazine	3 gm	Oral, initial dose subsequent doses up to 4 gm daily in divided doses.	A sulphonamide used in the treatment of systemic infections.
Sulphadimidine	3 gm	Initial dose, subsequent doses up to 6 gm daily in divided doses.	A sulphonamide used in the treatment of systemic infections.
	2 gm	Initial dose, subsequent doses up to 4 gm daily in divided doses.	In the treatment of urinary infections.
Testosterone	100 to 600 mg	By implantation.	Anabolic steroid.
Tetracycline hydrochloride	1 to 3 gm	Oral, daily in divided doses.	Broad spectrum antibiotic.
Thiamine hydrochloride (Vit. B_1)	2 to 5 mg	Oral, prophylactic dose.	A component of vitamin B complex.
	25 to 100 mg	Oral, daily therapeutic dose.	
	25 to 100 mg	By s/c or 1/m injection.	
Thyroid	30 to 250 mg	Oral, daily.	In hypothyroidism.
Tolbutamide	0.5 to 1.5 gm	Oral, daily.	In the treatment of mild diabetes.
Vasopressin injection	0.25 to 0.75 ml (5 to 15 units)	By s/c or 1/m injection.	In the treatment of diabetes.
Viomycin sulphate	0.5 to 1 mega unit	By 1/m injection daily or at longer intervals.	Antibiotic.

FACTORS AFFECTING DOSE OF A DRUG IN ANIMALS

1. Age

Young animals are more susceptible than adults therefore require less dose.

2. Body Weight and Size

The dose of a drug is determined more by the weight of the animal than by any other single factor, however, it must be borne in mind that weight is only an approximate determination of doses under many circumstances. Further study of doses in different species of animals and under different conditions within a species is necessary before deciding the actual dose of a drug.

The size of animals varies according to breeds. So, a dose which may be harmless for an animal of heavy breed may prove dangerous to animal of lighter breed. This is very important to remember in the case of dogs where one breed may be ten times heavier than the other breed.

3. Sex

The female of the species may require less dose than male. This may be due to lesser weight, pregnancy or lactation.

In female animals the doses of drugs must be adjusted according to the activity of reproductive organs. For example, during pregnancy strong purgatives should be avoided because of the hazard of inducing abortion. Some drugs have a tendency to pass into the milk which prevent its use for human consumption. Therefore such drugs must be used very carefully in milch cows.

4. Time of Administration

Time of administration of drugs is very important. Generally a small dose of a drug may be more effective when given in an empty stomach than when the same is given in full stomach. Anthelmintics and purgatives act better in empty stomach. Hypnotics are more effective if given at the end of the day rather than early in the morning.

Route of Administration

the same drug can be administered by all these routes the dose will vary the order given below :

oral > s/c > 1/m > 1/v

imatic Conditions

mperature and atmospheric moisture have a great influence on the of the animals. In a humid and hot climate less dose is required a dry and cold climate.

7. Surroundings and Work

Hypnotics may not produce sleep in noisy surroundings unless a heavier dose is administered. Well kept animals may bear a particular dose whereas the same dose may not be borne by ill kept animals.

8. Habit

An animal which is constantly under the influence of a drug may develop tolerance for that drug. The normal doses may fail to produce the desired effect and may require much bigger doses to get appreciable effect.

9. Species

The dose of a drug varies from species to species. The dose of a drug for a horse will be different from cow, from sheep, from goat, from pig, from dog, from cat, etc. Opium produces excitement in horse and cattle and narcosis in dog. These differences in action are due to anatomical and physiological peculiarities.

10. Synergistic or Antagonistic Effect

When two drugs having similar effect are given in the combined form the action is potentiated and a more powerful effect is produced than either of the individual drug even when given in equivalent dose.

Sometimes when two or more drugs are combined together, they oppose the effect of each other and ultimate therapeutic effect is decreased.

11. Character of the Drug

A crude drug has to be given in larger doses than its active principals or extracts. For example, nux vomica powder will have to be given in larger doses than its alkaloid strychnine.

12. Object of Medication

The dose of a drug varies with the purpose for which it is used. For example, magnesium sulphate act as purgative in large doses while in smaller doses it acts as laxative and antacid.

13. Rate of Elimination

The drugs which are excreted at a faster rate require larger doses than those drugs which are excreted at a slow rate.

Veterinary Doses

The following symbols or abbreviations are used :

H horse
C cow or cattle
D dog
Sh sheep

Name of drug	*Maximum dose*	*Route of administration*	*Uses*
Aluminium hydroxide gel	D : about 4 ml every 2 hr.	Oral.	Antacid.
Aminophylline	H : 2-5 gm t.i.d.	Orally for 2-3 weeks.	In broken wind in horses and to relieve bronchial spasm.
	D : 50-100 mg t.i.d. or q.i.d.	Orally, 1/v or 1/m.	
Ammonium chloride	H : 4-15 gm	Oral.	Urine acidifier.
	C : 15-30 gm		
	D : 0.2-0.5 gm		
	Sh : 1-2 gm		
Amphetamine	H, C : 100-300 mg	s/c	C.N.S. stimulant.
	D : 1.1-4.4 mg/kg	s/c or 1/m.	
Ampicillin	2-7 mg/kg body wt.	Parenteral.	Broad spectrum antibiotic.
	4-10 mg/kg body wt.	Oral.	
Aspirin	H : 30-47.5 mg/kg every 12 hrs.	Orally.	Analgesic.
	C : 100 mg/kg every 12 hrs.	Orally.	
	D : 10 mg/kg every 12 hrs.	Orally.	
	Cat : 10 mg/kg at 48 hrs. interval	Orally.	
Atropine sulphate	All species 0.045 mg/kg	s/c	Spasmolytic.
	0.5 to 1.0% soln.	Topical.	Mydriatic.
Barbital sodium	D : 0.15-1.0 gm	Oral.	Sedative.

(Contd.)

Name of drug	Maximum dose	Route of administration	Uses
	Cat : 0.1-0.3 gm		
Bemegride	D, Cat : 15-20 mg/kg	1/v	C.N.S. stimulant.
Benzyl penicillin	12,000 I.U./kg	1/m.	Antibiotic.
Caffeine and sodium benzoate	H, C : 5-10 gm	s/c, 1/m.	C.N.S. stimulant.
	Sh : 0.5-3 gm		
	D : 0.1-1.0 gm		
	Cat : 0.05-0.2 gm		
Calcium carbonate	H : 30-120 gm	Oral.	Antacid.
	C : 100-300 gm		
	Sh : 8-15 gm		
	D : 0.5-4.0 gm		
	Cat : 0.3-1.5 gm		
Castor oil	H, C : 250-1000 ml	Oral.	Cathartic.
	Sh : 50-150 ml		
	D : 5-25 ml		
	Cat : 3-15 ml		
Chloral hydrate	H, C, Sh : 40-100 mg/kg	Oral.	Sedative.
Chloramphenicol	H, C : 2-4 mg/kg	1/m.	Broad spectrum antibiotic.
	Sh, goat, calves, pigs : 4-10 mg/kg	1/m.	
	D : 165 mg/kg t.i.d.	Oral.	
	Cat : 0.25 gm once or twice daily	Oral.	
Chlorpromazine	Large animals : 1-2 mg/kg	1/m.	Tranquilizer, antiemetic. It is also used as an anticonvulsant and in treatment of colic in horses.
	0.5-1 mg/kg	1/v.	
	D, cat : 1.1-6.6 mg/kg	1/m.	
	0.55-4.4 mg/kg	1/v.	

(Contd.)

Name of drug	Maximum dose	Route of administration	Uses
Chlortetracycline hydrochloride	Large animals : 10-20 mg/kg/day given in two equally divided doses at 12 hours interval. Small animals : 25-50 mg/kg/day	Oral.	Broad spectrum antibiotic.
Cloxacillin	H, C : 1-2 mg/kg Small animals : 4-10 mg/kg	Parenteral.	Broad spectrum antibiotic.
Codeine phosphate	D : 1.1-2.2 mg/kg t.i.d. or q.i.d.	Oral.	Analgesic, antitussive, antidiarrhoeal.
Copper sulphate	1% solution Pig : 50-100 ml D, cat : 10-50 ml	Oral.	Emetic.
Diazepam	D, cat : 1 mg/kg (maximum 20 mg 1/v and 5 mg orally) Pig : 5.5 mg/kg	1/v or oral. 1/m.	Sedative, tranquilizer and anticonvulsant.
Digitalis powder	H : 33-66 mg/kg	Oral.	Used in congestive heart failure.
Digitalis tincture	H : 0.33-0.66 ml/kg	Oral.	Used in congestive heart failure.
Ephedrine	D : 15-30 mg b.i.d. or t.i.d.	Oral.	Bronchodialator, nasal decongestant, antidote in morphine and barbiturate overdosage.
Ergometrine maleate	H, C : 10-20 mg Sh, goat : 0.5-1 mg D : 0.2-1 mg Cat : up to 0.125 mg	Oral, parenteral. Oral, parenteral. Oral, parenteral. Oral, parenteral.	Used for expulsion of foetus and foetal membranes. Also used for prophylaxis and treatment of post-partum haemorrhage.

(Contd.)

Name of drug	*Maximum dose*	*Route of administration*	*Uses*
Erythromycin estolate	D, cat : 6.6-8.8 mg/kg/day in 3 or 4 divided doses.	Oral.	Bacteriostatic or bactericidal, effective against gram-positive organisms.
Ferrous sulphate	H : 2-8 gm C : 8-15 gm Sh : 0.5-2 gm D : 0.06-0.3 gm Cat : 0.03-0.2 gm	Oral.	Iron deficiency anaemia.
Gentamycin	D, cat : 2-4 mg/kg body wt. 2 times a day on the first day, once daily thereafter	1/m or s/c.	Broad spectrum antibiotic.
Griseofulvin	H : 100 mg/kg daily for 20 days Calf : 20-30 mg/kg D, cat : 7-20 mg/kg	Oral.	Antifungal antibiotic.
Hydrocortisone acetate	H, C : 1-15 gm 50-250 mg D : 2.2 mg/kg divided in 3 or 4 doses if given orally.	1/m. Intra-articular. 1/m.	Corticosteroid.
Insulin	D : initial dose may vary between 5-15 units/day depending on the severity of disease.	s/c	Diabetes mellitus.
Iron-dextran complex	Suckling pig : 2 ml of 5% soln. (100 mg)	1/m	Iron deficiency anaemia.
Kanamycin	15 mg/kg/day in 3 divided doses 20-30 mg/kg/day in 3-4 divided doses	1/m Oral.	Broad spectrum antibiotic.
Lead arsenate	Lamb : 0.5-1.0 gm Sh : 1.0 gm	Oral.	Anticestodal

(*Contd.*)

Name of drug	Maximum dose	Route of administration	Uses
	Calf : 0.5-1.0 gm		
	C : 2.0 gm		
Lidocaine hydrochloride	H, C : 10-20 ml of 2% soln.	s/c	As infiltration
(also known as	Pig, Sh : 8-12 ml of 2% soln.		anaesthetic.
Lignocaine hydrochloride)	D, cat : 1 ml of 2% soln./4.5 kg		For epidural anaesthesia.
	Goat : 0.2-0.4 ml/kg		
Lincomycin	D, cat : 20 mg/kg	1/m or s/c	Broad spectrum
	20 mg/kg b.i.d.	Oral.	antibiotic. Active against
	Pigs : 20 mg/kg once or twice daily	1/v	gram-positive
	10 mg/kg for 3-7 days	1/m	microorganisms.
Linseed oil	H : 500-750 ml	Oral.	Cathartic.
	C : 500-1000 ml		
	Sh : 25-100 ml		
	Pig : 50-150 ml		
Liquid paraffin	H, C : 250-1000 ml	Oral.	Cathartic.
	Sh : 25-150 ml		
	Pig : 25-300 ml		
	D : 5-30 ml		
	Cat : 2-6 ml		
Magnesium sulphate	H, C : 250-1000 gm	Oral.	Cathartic.
	Foal, calf : 25-50 gm		
	Sh : 25-125 gm		
	D : 5-25 gm		
	Cat : 2-5 gm		
Mebendazole	H : 10-15 mg/kg	Oral.	Anthelmintic.
	D, cat : 25 mg/kg for 5 days		

(Contd.)

Name of drug	Maximum dose	Route of administration	Uses
Mepridine HCl (Pethidine)	All species : 3-5 mg/kg	Oral or 1/m.	Analgesic.
	Cat : 11-22 mg/kg	1/v	
	D : 4.4 mg/kg	1/m	
Meprobamate	D : 400 mg t.i.d. or q.i.d.	Oral.	Sedative, hypnotic.
Methadone HCl	H : 0.12 mg/kg	1/v	Pre-anaesthetic use.
	H : 0.25 mg/kg	1/m or s/c	As an analgesic.
	D : 1.1 mg/kg	Oral or s/c	
Morphine sulphate	0.12 mg/kg	1/v	Spasmodic colic in horses.
	0.22 mg/kg	1/m or slow 1/v injection in acute cases.	
	D : 0.1-2 mg/kg	s/c	For pre-anaesthetic medication.
	Cat : 0.1 mg/kg	s/c	
	Pig : 0.2-0.9 mg	s/c	
Nalorphine HCl	D : 2 mg/kg	s/c	As an antidote for opium alkaloids.
Neomycin sulphate	H, C : 4-7.5 gm	Oral.	Intestinal antiseptic.
	Foal, calves 2-3 gm		
	Lambs, piglets : 0.75-1.0 gm		
	D : 0.2-0.5 gm. May be divided in 2-4 doses		
Nikethamide	As 25% injectable solution		
	H, C : 10-20 ml	1/m or 1/v	Respiratory stimulant.
	D : 1-3 ml	1/m or 1/v	
	Cat : 0.5-2.0 ml	1/m or 1/v	
Nitrofurantoin	D : 2-10 mg/kg 6-8 hourly for 7-14 days.	Oral.	Urinary antiseptic.

(*Contd.*)

Name of drug	Maximum dose	Route of administration	Uses
	3.3 mg/kg b.i.d.	1/m	
Novobiocin	Fowl and turkeys : 2-3.5 gm/9 kg feed	Oral.	Narrow spectrum antibiotic.
Nystatin	D : 22,000 I.U./kg	Oral.	Antifungal antibiotic.
Oxytetracycline HCl	Foal, calf : 10-20 mg/kg Pig : 10-30 mg/kg D, cat : 27 mg/kg b.i.d. Poultry : 10-60 gm/100 kg feed or 0.1-0.3 gm/litre of water	Oral.	Broad spectrum antibiotic.
Oxytocin	1/m injection — 1/v injection H, C : 10-40 I.U. — 2.5-10 I.U. Sh, goat, pig : 2.5-10 I.U. — 0.5-2.5 I.U. D : 1-10 I.U. — up to 0.5 I.U. Cat : 0.5-5 I.U. — — 1/v dose should be diluted to 1 : 10 with dextrose or distilled water.		Used to produce contraction in uterus. It is also used for 'letting down' of milk.
Penicillin	All species : 11,000 I.U./kg	1/m	Antibiotic.
Phenazone (Antipyrin)	H : 8-16 gm C : 12-24 gm Sh, pig : up to 2 gm D : 0.3-0.6 gm	Oral.	Antipyretic.
Phenobarbitone sodium	D : 30-300 mg	Oral.	For sedation and hypnosis.
	Cat : 15-60 mg D : 2.2 mg/kg 2-3 times daily		As an anticonvulsant.
Phenolphthalein	D, cat : 10 mg/kg	Oral.	Purgative.
Picrotoxin	D : 1-3 mg	1/v	C.N.S. stimulant.

(*Contd.*)

Name of drug	*Maximum dose*	*Route of administration*	*Uses*
Piprazine adipate	H : 10 gm/45 kg body weight (maximum dose 60 gm); repeat at an interval of 2 months.	Oral.	Anthelmintic.
	C : 10 gm/45 kg body weight; repeat as required.		
	Sh, goat : 3-5 gm in feed		
	D, cat : 0.1 gm/kg body weight in feed		
	Pig : 0.2 gm/kg body weight		
Prednisolone acetate	D : up to 25 mg	Oral.	Antiketosis.
	Cat : 0.5-1.0 mg b.i.d.		
Prednisone	H, C : 100-300 mg	1/m	Antiketosis.
	H, C : 50-250 mg	1/articularly	Anti-inflammatory.
	Dog : 0.5-2 mg/kg	Oral, 1/m	
Promazine HCl	H : 0.44-1.1 mg/kg	1/m or 1/v	Anti-emetic and in pre-anaesthetic medication.
	H, C : 1.65-2.75 mg/kg	Oral.	
	Pig : 2 mg/kg	1/m	
	D : 2-6 mg/kg	1/m or 1/v	
Quinidine sulphate	D : 6-20 mg/kg every 6-8 hours	Orally.	In the treatment of arterial fibrillation in dogs and horses.
	2-6 mg/kg	1/m	
Secobarbital	D, cat : 30-200 mg (depending on purpose and size of the animal)	Oral.	Short acting hypnotic and sedative.
Sodium bromide	H : 25-50 gm	Oral.	Sedative.
	Pig : 5-10 gm		
	D : 0.3-3.0 gm		

(*Contd.*)

Name of drug	Maximum dose	Route of administration	Uses
	Cat : 0.06-0.3 gm		
Sodium Salicylate	H, C : 15-20 gm	Oral.	Analgesic.
	Sh, pig : 1-4 gm		
	D : 0.3-1.0 gm		
	Cat : 0.1-0.3 gm		
Streptomycin sulphate	H : 5-10 mg/kg body weight every 3-4 hours	1/m	Antibiotic (effective against gram-negative bacteria).
	C, calf : 10-15 mg/kg every 12-24 hours	1/m	
	Pig, Sh : 5-10 mg/kg every 3-4 hours	1/m	
	D, cat : 10-20 mg/kg every 8-12 hours	1/m	
Strychnine sulphate	H, C : 15-60 mg	s/c	Stimulant.
	Sh : 5-15 mg	s/c	
	Pig : 2-8 mg	s/c	
	D : 0.3-1.0 mg	s/c	
	Cat : 0.1-0.5 mg	s/c	
Tetracycline	H, C, Sh, pig : 2.2-4.4 mg/kg	1/m	Broad spectrum antibiotic.
	D, cat : 4.4-11 mg/kg	1/m	
Trimethoprim and sulpha	Large animals : 30 mg/kg body weight	Oral.	Bactericidal.
	Small animals : 15 mg/kg body weight daily for 5 days		
	Cats : 120 mg daily		

VETERINARY PRESCRIPTIONS

Rx

Liquid extract of belladonna	2 ml
Potassium iodide	4 gm
Glycerin	30 ml
Water	60 ml

Fiat mistura for a cattle. Mitte doses quarta.
Sig : Unus b.i.d. more dicto sumenda.

Procedure

Dissolve potassium iodide in small amount of water. To this add liquid extract of belladonna and glycerin. Mix thoroughly and add remaining amount of water with continuous stirring until uniform.

Rx

Potassium chlorate	0.5 gm
Tincture ipecac	1.0 ml
Syrup scilla	2.0 ml
Water q.s.	10.0 ml

Fiat mistura for a dog. Mitte doses quinque.
Sig : Unus t.i.d. sumenda.

Procedure

Dissolve potassium chlorate in water. To this add tincture ipecac and syrup scilla with continuous stirring until a uniform mixture is obtained.

Rx

Sodium salicylate	250 mg
Sodium bicarbonate	150 mg
Simple syrup	2 ml
Water q.s.	15 ml

Fiat mistura for a dog. Mitte tales novem.
Sig : 15 ml t.d.s.

Procedure

Dissolve sodium salicylate in water. To this dissolve sodium bicarbonate and add simple syrup. Stir thoroughly so as to get a uniform mixture.

Rx

Ammonium bromide	6 gm
Sodium bromide	6 gm
Potassium bromide	6 gm

Syrup q.s.	150 ml

Fiat mistura for a dog.
Sig : 5-15 ml omni quarta hora.

Procedure

Dissolve ammonium bromide, sodium bromide and potassium bromide in sufficient syrup. Mix thoroughly and then add more of syrup to produce the required volume.

Rx

Chloral hydrate	30 gm
Linseed oil	ad 500 ml

Fiat haustus.
Sig : Statim sumat. Rep. s.o.s.

Procedure

Dissolve chloral hydrate in linseed oil with continuous stirring.

Rx

Sodium bicarbonate	4 gm
Tincture nux vomica	1 ml
Tincture gentian co.	6 ml
Simple syrup	15 ml
Peppermint water q.s.	90 ml

Fiat mistura for a dog. Mitte 180 ml.
Sig : 15 ml t.d.s.

Procedure

Dissolve sodium bicarbonate in about 45 ml peppermint water. To this add tincture nux vomica, tincture gentian co. and simple syrup one by one with continuous stirring. Add more of peppermint water to produce the required volume.

Rx

Chloral hydrate	20 gm
Turpentine oil	30 ml
Linseed oil q.s.	500 ml

Fiat haustus for a horse.
Sig : Statim sumat.

Procedure

Dissolve chloral hydrate in sufficient linseed oil. To this incorporate turpentine oil and add more of linseed oil to produce the required volume.

Rx

Magnesium sulphate	25 gm
Magnesium carbonate	4 gm
Peppermint water q.s.	180 ml

Fiat mistura. Mitte 90 ml.
Sig : 15 ml pro dose.

Procedure

Mix magnesium sulphate and magnesium carbonate in a mortar. Measure out ¾th of the vehicle. Out of this add small amount of vehicle to the mixed powders and triturate thoroughly so as to produce a thick cream. Then add the remainder amount of measured out vehicle with continuous trituration. Add more of vehicle to produce the required volume.

Rx

Ferrous sulphate	40 gm
Tannic acid	4 gm
Strong tincture of ginger	30 ml
Water q.s.	500 ml

Fiat mistura for a large animal.
Sig : Give 150 ml once daily in 500 ml of rice gruel until the diarrhoea ceases.

Procedure

Dissolve ferrous sulphate in about 200 ml water. Separately dissolve tannic acid in 100 ml water. Mix the two and add strong tincture of ginger. Add more of vehicle to produce the required volume.

Rx

Potassium tartrate	0.5 gm
Sodium bicarbonate	0.5 gm
Magnesium sulphate	1.0 gm

Fiat pulvis for a dog. Mitte tales quarta.
Sig : Give twice a day with food.

Procedure

Mix potassium tartrate, sodium bicarbonate and magnesium sulphate thoroughly in a pestle and mortar. Wrap in a powder paper.

Rx

Light magnesium carbonate	6	gm
Kaolin	2	gm
Ipecac powder	0.5	gm

Fiat pulvis. Mitte tales sexies.

Sig : Ter in die sumenda.

Procedure

Mix light magnesium carbonate, kaolin and ipecac powder in a mortar. Triturate thoroughly so as to get a uniform powder. Divide into required number of powders and wrap in powder papers.

Rx

Chloral hydrate	30 gm
Gur q.s.	

Fiat bolus (balls) for horse. Mitte tales duo.

Sig : Give one bolus at once. Repeat, if necessary, at an interval of two hours.

Procedure

Mix chloral hydrate with gur thoroughly in a mortar so as to get a uniform mass. Divide the mixed material into two parts and prepare bolus. Wrap in powder papers.

Revision Questions

I. Very short answer type questions

Answer the following questions in brief.

(a) What is 'Posology'?

(b) Define 'Dose'.

(c) Name the formulas by which the dose for a child can be calculated from adult dose.

(d) What happens if the drug is administered lesser than the prescribed dose or higher than the proscribed dose?

II. Short answer type questions

Explain the following :

(i) Young's rule

(ii) Dilling's rule

(iii) Clark's formula

(iv) Accumulation

(v) Synergism

(vi) Antagonism
(vii) Habituation
(viii) Addiction
(ix) Idiosyncrasy
(x) Hypersensitivity
(xi) Tolerance
(xii) Tachyphylaxis.

III. Long answer type questions

1. Explain the term 'Dose'. Discuss various factors which affect the dose of a drug.
2. Describe various methods by which the child dose of a drug can be calculated from adult dose.
3. Discuss different factors which affect the dose of a drug in animals.
4. Give the dose, route of administration and used of the following drugs :

(i) Adrenaline injection
(ii) Ampicillin
(iii) Ascorbic acid
(iv) Aspirin
(v) B.C.G. vaccine
(vi) Caffeine
(vii) Calciferol
(viii) Castor oil
(ix) Chloral hydrate
(x) Chloramphenicol
(xi) Codeine phosphate
(xii) Cod liver oil
(xiii) Diazepam
(xiv) Emetine hydrochloride
(xv) Erythromycin
(xvi) Ferrous sulphate
(xvii) Folic acid
(xviii) Gentamycin sulphate
(xix) Griseofulvin
(xx) Isoniazid
(xxi) Light kaolin
(xxii) Light magnesium carbonate
(xxiii) Liquid paraffin
(xxiv) Magnesium sulphate
(xxv) Morphine sulphate
(xxvi) Nux vomica tincture

(xxvii) Oxytetracycline hydrochloride
(xxviii) Paracetamol
(xxix) Paraldehyde
(xxx) Phenacetin
(xxxi) Phenobarbitone sodium
(xxxii) Pethidine hydrochloride
(xxxiii) Prednisone
(xxxiv) Quinine sulphate
(xxxv) Sodium bicarbonate
(xxxvi) Sodium salicylate
(xxxvii) Streptomycin sulphate
(xxxviii) Testosterone
(xxxix) Tetracycline hydrochloride
(xl) Tolbutamide

4

Powders

Powders are the solid dosage form of medicament which are meant for internal and external use. They are available in crystalline or amorphous form. Though the drugs are prepared in many different physical forms and shapes but many of them are prepared by using powders in one way or the other. Each dosage form so prepared has certain advantages over the other form. Similarly, the powders have certain advantages as described below :

1. Most of the drugs are available in powder forms and it becomes more convenient for the physician to prescribe specific amount of medicament according to the need of the patient.
2. Powders are usually more stable than liquids because chemical reactions take place more rapidly in atmospheric conditions when the drug is in liquid dosage form than powder.
3. Incompatibility is less in case of powders than liquids.
4. The smaller particle size of powders produces more rapid dissolution in the body fluids than other solid dosage forms of medicament, e.g., tablets, capsules or pills. The rapid dissolution increases the blood concentration in a shorter time, thereby the action is produced in a lesser time.
5. Large quantities of bulky drugs which are otherwise difficult to administer can be easily administered by mixing with liquids.
6. They are more easy to carry than liquids.
7. They are more economical as compared to other dosage forms because for extemporaneous preparation they do not require any special technique or machinery.
8. Children and old persons who cannot swallow solid dosage forms can easily injest powders which can be dispersed in water or any other liquid and may be administered through feeding tube to the patients who are fed by tubes which terminate in the stomach itself.

Disadvantage

1. Drugs which deteriorate on exposure to atmospheric conditions are not suitable for dispensing in powder forms.
2. Bitter, nauseous, corrosive and unpalatable drugs cannot be dispensed in powder form.

3. Deliquescent and hygroscopic drugs cannot be dispensed in powder form.
4. Volatile drugs are not suitable for dispensing in powder form.

CLASSIFICATION OF POWDERS

1. Simple and compound powders for internal use (Divided Powders).
2. Granular effervescent powders for internal use.
3. Bulk powders for external use, e.g., dusting powders, insufflations and tooth powders, etc.
4. Powders enclosed in catchets and capsules.
5. Compressed powders (Tablets) and tablet triturates.

Simple and Compound Powders

Simple Powders

A simple powder contains only one ingredient either in crystalline or amorphous form. When the powder is in the crystalline form, preferably it is reduced to fine powder, weighed and wrapped as individual doses as described in compound powders.

Rx

Aspirin 300 mg

Fiat pulvis. Mitte tales quarta.

Rx

Calcium gluconate 1 gm

Make powder. Send such six.

Compound Powders

Compound powders contain two or more than two substances which are mixed together and then divided into individual doses.

Rx

Aspirin	300 mg
Paracetamol	150 mg
Caffeine	50 mg

Fiat pulvis. Mitte tales octo.
Sig : Unus dolore urgente sumenda.
Type : Oral divided powder.

General Method of Preparation

Since there is little unavoidable loss of powder during weighing and mixing because some powder will adhere to the spatula, pestle and the mortar therefore calculate for one extra powder than required, but if by calculating for one extra powder an awkward fraction of weights is involved then a suitable number of extra powders may be calculated.

The dispensing balances are not so sensitive that the quantities less than 2 grain or 130 mg can be weighed accurately therefore the quantities weighing less than 2 grain or 130 mg must be triturated with a suitable inert diluent so that the quantities are made weighable on dispensing balance. Generally lactose is used as a diluent because it is colourless, soluble and compatible with majority of drugs. It is preferred to sucrose because sucrose has tendency to absorb moisture and become a cake.

Separately powder a slight excess of each crystalline substance. Weight out the required amount of each powder and diluent, i.e., lactose, if necessary. Mix all the ingredients in the ascending order of their weights and mix thoroughly so that a homogenous powder is formed.

Weigh out the required number of powders and wrap in the papers.

The volatile substances and hygroscopic powders require to be double wrapped, the inner wrapper of which should be of wax paper to prevent volatilization and absorption of moisture.

Marketed Powders

1. Acidin with belladonna powder (East India Pharmaceutical Works, Calcutta - 700071).
2. Bismag powder (Geoffrey Manners & Co. Ltd., Bombay - 400038).

   Contains :

   Sod. bicarbonate, heavy magnesium carbonate, light magnesium carbonate, calcium carbonate.
3. Prequest powder (sachet) [Parke-Davis (India) Ltd., Bombay - 400025].

   Contains :

Sod. chloride	0.365%
Sod. acid phos.	0.975%
Sod. citrate	1.839%
Pot. chloride	2.330%
Mag. sulphate	0.736%
Cal. lactate	0.545%
Dextrose anhydrous	89.900%

4. Raylyte powder (Rays Laboratories Pvt. Ltd., Calcutta - 700007).

   Each 27.5 gm contains :

Sod. chloride	3.5 gm
Sod. bicarbonate	2.5 gm
Pot. chloride	1.5 gm
Dextrose	20.0 gm

5. Takazyme powder [Parke-Davis (India) Ltd., Bombay - 400025].

Each contains :
Mag. carbonate light 16%
Mag. trisilicate 8%
Aspergillus (oryzae enzyme equ. to 1.07% alpha amylase)

POWDERS REQUIRING SPECIAL CONSIDERATIONS

1. Hygroscopic and Deliquescent Powders

Substances which absorb moisture from the atmosphere are not suitable for dispensing in powder papers because the absorbed moisture may promote the chemical degradation of the drug and in the case of effervescent preparations the acids may completely react with sodium bicarbonate rendering the preparation unfit for use. Among the commonly prescribed hygroscopic and deliquescent substances are ammonium chloride, ammonium bromide, ammonium iodide, calcium chloride, hyoscine hydrobromide, iron and ammonium citrate, pepsin, phenobarbitone sodium, potassium citrate, sodium bromide, sodium iodide, citric and tartaric acid.

When dispensing such powders, there are several precautions which a pharmacist must take to minimise absorption of moisture from the atmosphere. In first place the hygroscopic substances are usually supplied in granular form in order to expose less surface area to the atmosphere. These powders should not be finely powdered. If the need arises then the powdering may be carried out in a mortar which has been dried and warmed. Such powders should be double wrapped. In humid weather or when dealing with very deliquescent substances further wrapping in aluminium foil or plastic cover is advisable.

2. Eutectic Mixtures

When two or more substances are mixed together they liquefy due to the formation of a new compound which has a lower melting point than room temperature. The degree of liquefaction of eutectic substances is governed by their melting points, relative proportions and room temperature. The formation of eutectic mixtures signifies a physical change rather than a chemical change. The substances which on mixing liquefy are : menthol, acetanilide, thymol, phenacetin, camphor, aspirin, phenol, antipyrine, salol, chloral hydrate.

In dealing with eutectic substances firstly they may be dispensed as separate set of powders with directions that one set of each kind shall be taken as a dose. Secondly they may be incorporated in powders by adding an inert absorbent like magnesium carbonate, light magnesium oxide, kaolin, starch, lactose, calcium phosphate, bentonite, etc. Generally an equal amount of absorbent as that of eutectic substance is sufficient to prevent liquefaction. In this method each eutectic substance is mixed with an absorbent separately and then blended together lightly with a spatula on a sheet of paper. On the other hand when the substances which liquefy are present in small amount they may be mixed together so as to form a eutectic mixture, then the liquid so formed is absorbed by adding an absorbent. The remaining ingredients of the prescription are then incorporated and mixed together.

Rx

Menthol	5 gm
Camphor	5 gm
Ammonium chloride	30 gm
Light magnesium carbonate	60 gm

Fiat insufflatio. Mitte 50 gm.

Sig : Pro naso.

Type : Compound powder containing liquefiable substances.

3. Efflorescent Powders

Crystalline substances liberate water of crystallization wholly or partly due to change in relative humidity or during trituration, causing the powder to become wet or to liquefy. This difficulty may be overcome by using either corresponding anhydrous salt or an inert substance may be mixed with efflorescent substance before incorporating the other ingredients.

4. Vegetable Powders

Vegetable powders which contain volatile oils should not be subjected to heavy grinding in a mortar. When it is necessary to powder them, they must be powdered lightly in a mortar to prevent the loss of volatile oils present in them. In dispensing such vegetable powders and other volatile substances they must be double wrapped, inner wrapper of which should be of wax paper.

5. Liquids

If the quantity of the liquid to be incorporated is small, it may be triturated with an equal amount of powder, then the rest of the ingredients are incorporated in small portions with continuous trituration. If the quantities of liquids are large then an absorbent must be added.

Tinctures and fluid extracts will have to be evaporated but they should not be evaporated directly to dryness or a hard resinous mass which may be difficult to remove from the dish as well as difficult to mix with other ingredients. Therefore they must be partially evaporated until the liquid attains a syrupy consistency. Add lactose or any other suitable diluent and continue evaporation to dryness. Then incorporate other ingredients. The diluent is added to prevent the formation of sticky mass on evaporation. Whenever possible it is preferable to use powdered extracts instead of tinctures and fluid extracts in prescriptions.

6. Explosive Substances

When an oxidising agent and reducing agent are triturated in a mortar there are chances of explosion which may lead to serious consequences. Though the prescriptions for such combinations in powder form are rare, preferably should not be filled but if it has to be dispensed then powder each ingredient separately in a mortar and mix them lightly with other ingredients. Alternatively powder each substance separately and dispense them in separate powder paper with suitable directions to the patient regarding its use.

List of Oxidising and Reducing Agents

Oxidising agents	*Reducing agents*
Potassium chlorate	Charcoal
Potassium dichromate	Sulphur
Potassium nitrate	Sulphides
Potassium permanganate	Tannic acid
Silver nitrate	

Rx

Potassium chlorate	600 mg
Tannic acid	300 mg
Sucrose	300 mg

Fiat charta. Mitte tales tres.

Signa : Unus aqua cyathus gargarisma.

7. Potent Drugs

Substances having a maximum dose of less than one grain and poisonous substances should be regarded as potent substances. Small quantities of potent drugs should not be weighed on dispensing balance. The best method is to prepare triturations. These are dilutions of potent powdered drugs, prepared by intimate mixing of the drug with suitable diluent in definite proportion. In this method the drug is reduced to fine powder and to this an equal amount of diluent is mixed well by thorough trituration in a mortar. To this is incorporated the rest of the diluent in successive portions with thorough trituration each time until whole of the diluent has been added. Under no circumstances the whole of the diluent should be added to the drug at one time otherwise the potent drug will not be mixed uniformly and thoroughly in the diluent resulting in uneven dose in divided powders.

Rx

Prednisone 8 mg

Send such four powders.

Signa : One to be taken as directed.
Type: Simple divided potent powder.

Rx

Phenobarbitone sodium 15 mg

Send such 4 powders.
Sig : Unus omni nocte sumenda.
Type : Simple oral divided potent powder.

8. Granular Powders

Sometimes it is difficult to present solid medicaments with large doses in suitable dosage form. The tablets and capsules cannot be prescribed because a large number of them will be required to take as a single dose which is not feasible, liquids cannot be prepared because of stability problems. Therefore the choice remains to powders. But the bitter, nauseous and unpleasant powders are difficult to dispense as such, therefore these powders are prepared in the form of granules.

On a small scale the medicaments are mixed with sweetening, flavouring and colouring agents in a mortar. A suitable granulating agent is added to moisten the powders until the mass becomes coherent but not too damp. The granulating agents used may be water, starch mucilage, gelatin or sugar solutions and various dilutions of alcohol. Press down the coherent mass through sieve number 10 superimposed on sieve number 20 or 24. Dry the granules by spreading in a warm place for 2-3 hours or by keeping them in an oven at a temperature not exceeding 60°C. Pack them in dry, well closed, wide mouthed bottles.

On a large scale manufacturing various types of granulators are used for preparing the granules.

Now a days some of the antibiotics like erythromycin, nystatin, phenoxymethyl penicillin, etc., which are unstable in solution are prepared in the dry granular form in which the drug is mixed with suspending, sweetening, flavouring, colouring and granulating agents. The granules are prepared and packed as usual. The bottle is labelled with the instructions that the patient should add specified amount of freshly boiled and cooled water to granules. The bottle should be shaken well so as to form a homogeneous solution. The label should also carry the storage conditions and time limit in which the reconstituted preparation should be consumed.

Marketed Granules

1. Antepar granules [Burroughs Wellcome (India) Ltd., Bombay - 400023].

   Each contains :

   Piperazine citrate equ. to 4.5 gm of piperazine hexahydrate and cal. sennosides equ. to 12 mg of sennosides A & B.

2. Calcirol granules (Cadila Labs Ltd., Ahmedabad - 380050).

   Each gm contains :
   Vitamin D_3 60,000 I.U.

3. Flush granules (Dey's Medical Stores, Calcutta - 700087).

   Each 5 gm contains :

Isabgul husk	3.25	gm
Baked bael	0.9	gm
Myrobalan	0.2	gm
Guar gum	0.35	gm

4. Protinex granules (Pfizer Ltd., Bombay - 400021).
   Multivitamin preparation.
5. Alprovit granules (Alkem Labs Ltd., Bombay - 400018).
   Multivitamin preparation.

Marketed Dry Syrups

1. Amfimox dry syrup [Toshniwal Drugs & Pharmaceuticals (P) Ltd. New Delhi - 110002].

   Each 5 ml contains :
   Amoxycillin 125 mg.

2. Ampark dry syrup [Parke-Davis (India) Ltd., Bombay - 400025].

   Each 5 ml contains :
   Ampicillin 125 mg.

3. Ceff dry syrup (Lupin Labs Ltd., Bombay - 400098).

   Each 5 ml contains :
   Cephalexin 125 mg, 250 mg.

4. E-mycin granules (Themis Pharmaceuticals, Bombay - 400093).

   Each 5 ml contains :
   Erythromycin 100 mg.

5. Moxydil dry syrup (Duphar-Interfran Ltd., Bombay - 400018).

   Each 5 ml contains :
   Amoxycillin trihydrate 125 mg, 250 mg.

6. Penmix dry syrup (Deepharma Ltd., New Delhi - 110020).

   Each 3 gm contains :
   Ampicillin 125 mg
   Cloxacillin 125 mg

EFFERVESCENT GRANULES

Effervescent granules are the specially prepared solid dosage form of medicament, meant for internal use. They usually contain a soluble medicinal agent mixed with citric acid, tartaric acid, and sodium bicarbonate. Before administration they are suspended, dissolved in water or are mixed with soft drinks. On mixing with water the carbon dioxide is released as a result of acid-base reaction producing effervescence and the mixture is taken while effervescing. The carbonated water produced from the release of carbon dioxide serves to mask the saline and bitter taste of drugs and the carbon dioxide is said to stimulate the flow of gastric juice and accelerate absorption of medicament.

Effervescent granules are preferred to effervescent powders in order to decrease the rate of dissolution of the substances upon addition to water. Further, if powders are used there may be violent and uncontrollable effervescence with loss of carbon dioxide and ultimately the carbonation of solution may decrease to a great extent.

Method of Preparation

The ingredients used for the preparation of effervescent granules consist of sodium bicarbonate, citric acid, tartaric acid and sodium acid phosphate. Sodium acid phosphate is commonly used in commercial preparations because it is more economical than organic acids. Sodium bicarbonate is used to react with acids when the preparation is added to water, leading to evolution of carbon dioxide. The quantity of the acids used is slightly more than the quantity actually required for complete neutralization of sodium bicarbonate because the preparation with slightly acidic taste are more palatable. The tartaric acid is anhydrous whereas citric acid contains one molecule of water of crystallization which is liberated during heating and serves as a moistening agent for the powders during granulation.

$$3NaHCO_3 + \underset{\text{(Citric acid)}}{C_6H_8O_7 \cdot H_2O} = \underset{\text{(Sodium citrate)}}{C_6H_5Na_3O_7} + 3CO_2 + 3H_2O$$

$$2NaHCO_3 + \underset{\text{(Tartaric acid)}}{C_4H_6O_6} = \underset{\text{(Sodium tartrate)}}{C_4H_4Na_2O_6} + 2CO_2 + 2H_2O$$

Citric acid and tartaric acid both are used because if citric acid alone is used it contains one molecule of water of crystallization which is liberated on heating, will make the mass too wet which will be difficult to pass through the sieve. If tartaric acid alone is used, it is anhydrous and some non-solvent liquid would have to be used for the preparation of granules, otherwise the resulting granules would not be firm but will crumble readily and give salty taste. Moreover citric acid partially neutralizes sodium bicarbonate, the rest of sodium bicarbonate is neutralized by tartaric acid, the slight excess of which imparts acidic taste to the preparation. So relative proportions of citric acid and tartaric acid are based on quantity of water needed to make the powder coherent.

There are two methods of preparation of effervescent granules.

(i) Heat method

(ii) Wet method.

(i) Heat Method

A large porcelain or stainless steel evaporating dish is placed over water bath which is being heated to boiling point and must ensure that the evaporating dish is hot when the powders are added to it, failing to do so will not provide sufficient water needed for granulation which will be liberated by citric acid on heating. If the dish will not be hot when the powders are added, it will heat up slowly and the liberated water of crystallization will go on evaporating simultaneously and at no time sufficient water will be available to effect granulation. The water needed for granulation is provided from two sources : (i) from water of crystallization of citric acid which is liberated during heating; and (ii) the water produced from the reactions of citric acid and tartaric acid with sodium bicarbonate.

The powdered ingredients are passed through a sieve no. 60, weighed and mixed. Then they are placed in the dish already warmed on water bath and pressed down with a spatula until the mixture has formed a loose cake or a damp coherent mass is formed. The damp mass is then pressed down a sieve to prepare the granules and dried by keeping in an oven at a temperature not exceeding 60°C. They are packed in dry, wide mouth air-tight containers.

Formula for the preparation of 40 gm of Citro-tartrate of soda effervescent granular base :

Sodium bicarbonate powder	20.40 gm
Tartaric acid powder	10.80 gm
Citric acid powder	7.20 gm
Refined sugar powder	6.00 gm

The method of preparation is described in the above paragraph.

Loss of weight occurs during granulation from two factors :

(a) Loss of moisture by evaporation from the damp mixture.

(b) Loss of carbon dioxide in the above reactions.

These losses constitute approximately one-seventh of the weight of powder used and must be taken into consideration while calculating the amount of granules to be prepared.

(ii) Wet Method

In the wet method, the mixed ingredients are moistened with a suitable liquid (for which alcohol is the most suitable) in a dish in which alcohol is added in small portions with continuous stirring until a coherent mass is formed. The mass is then passed through a no. 6 sieve and the granules dried at a temperature not exceeding 60°C. The dried granules are again passed through the sieve to break the lumps which may have formed during drying, then they are packed in wide mouth air-tight containers.

Marketed Effervescent Powders

1. Eno fruit salt (Smith Kline Beecham, Nabha - 147201, Punjab).
2. Cetri-soda [Abbot Labs (India) Ltd., Bombay - 400070].
3. Rhino (Mehta Unani Pharmacy & Co., Rajkot - 360001, Gujarat).

Marketed Effervescent Tablets

1. Pepfiz (Ranbaxy Labs Ltd., Delhi - 110020).

BULK POWDERS

They are supplied in bulk quantities and the patient measures out the dose according to his need. The bulk powders meant for internal use are supplied in wide-mouthed containers in which a teaspoon can be entered for easy removal of the contents. Only the nonpotent substances are supplied as bulk powders, e.g., antacids, laxatives, etc.

Bulk powders meant for external application like antiseptic and dusting powders are supplied in cardboard, glass or plastic containers, which are often designed for the specific method of application. The dusting powders are preferably supplied in perforated or sifter top containers.

Rx

Calcium carbonate	37.5 gm
Heavy magnesium carbonate	37.5 gm
Sodium bicarbonate	12.5 gm
Bismuth carbonate	12.5 gm

Make a powder.
Label : The Compound Bismuth Powder. Send 50 gm.
Sig : 5 gm bis in die sumenda.
Type : Bulk powder.

Rx

Rhubarb, in powder	25.0 gm
Ginger, in powder	10.0 gm
Light magnesium carbonate	32.5 gm
Heavy magnesium carbonate	32.5 gm

Make powder.
Label : The Gregory's powder (Compound Rhubarb powder). Send 25 gm.
Directions : 0.5 to 5.0 gm to be taken twice in a day.
Type : Bulk oral powder.

DUSTING POWDERS

Dusting powders are meant for external application to the skin for antiseptic, antipruritic, astringent, antiperspirant, absorbent, protective and lubricant purposes. These powders must be homogenous and in a very fine state of subdivision to enhance effectiveness and minimise local irritation. For this purpose they may be passed through a sieve no. 120. Additionally the dusting powders should flow easily, spread uniformly and stick to the skin when applied. They must be able to protect the skin from irritation caused by friction, moisture or chemical irritants.

Dusting powders are generally prepared by mixing two or more than two ingredients in which starch, kaolin or talc is used as one of the ingredients of formulation. Starch being a carbohydrate can support bacterial growth therefore rarely used. Talcum and other similar substances though are chemically inert substances but are readily contaminated with microorganisms like clostridium tetani, cl. welchii and bacillus anthracis. Therefore they must be sterilized before using in the formulation otherwise they may be a source of infection.

The dusting powders are dispensed in sifter-top containers or pressure aerosols. The pressure aerosol containers are costlier than other containers but can protect the powder from atmospheric conditions and help in the easy application of the preparation. Dusting powders may also be applied with powder puff, a soft brush or a sterile gauze pad but care must be taken to avoid mechanical irritation to the skin surface.

Though the dusting powders are considered non-toxic but the inhalation of light, fluffy powders may lead to pulmonary inflammation of lungs in infants and absorption of boric acid through the broken skin may cause toxic reactions in infants. Therefore proper care must be taken while using these types of preparations.

Rx

Purified talc, sterilised	50 gm
Starch, in powder	25 gm
Zinc oxide	25 gm

Label : Zinc, Starch and Talc dusting powder.

Type : Dusting powder.

Theory

This preparation contains talc which is mineral ingredient and may be contaminated with spores of clostridium tetani and clostridium welchii (a source of tetanus). Therefore whenever talc and kaolin is to be used in dusting powders, must be sterilised by heating at 160°C for one hour to remove these microorganisms. Purified talc has excellent flow and lubricant properties therefore is used in a number of dusting powders. Starch acts as an absorbent. Zinc oxide acts as an antiseptic and absorbs moisture.

Boric acid should no longer be used in dusting powders since it has been found that it may be absorbed in large amounts through the open skin leading to toxic reactions.

Procedure

Weigh the required quantities of purified talc, sterilised; starch, in powder and zinc oxide. Mix zinc oxide with starch, incorporate purified talc, sterilized. Mix thoroughly. Pass the mixed powders through a sieve no. 120 to remove gritty particles. After sifting, whole of the powder must again be lightly mixed. Pack the powder in sifter-top containers to protect it from air, moisture and contamination as well as convenience of application.

Marketed Dusting Powders

1. Cibazol dusting powder (Hindustan Ciba-Geigy Ltd., Bombay - 400020).

   Contains :

Sulphathiazole	20% w/w

2. Nebasulf dusting powder (Pfizer Ltd., Bombay - 400021).

   Each gm contains :

Neomycin sulphate	5 mg
Bacitracin	250 units
Sulphacetamide	60 mg

3. Neobacid sprinkling powder [Roland Pharmaceuticals, Berhampur, Distt. Ganjam (Orissa) - 760009].

   Each gm contains :

Neomycin sulphate	5 mg
Bacitracin	250 units
Sulphacetamide	60 mg

4. Salicylic acid compound dusting powder (Alpine Industries, New Delhi - 110028).

   Each contains :

Salicylic acid	1.5 gm
Boric acid	2.5 gm
Purified talc to	50.0 gm

5. Boric talc dusting powder (Alpine Industries, New Delhi - 110028).

   Each contains :

Boric acid	2.5 gm
Starch	5.0 gm
Purified talc to	50.0 gm

INSUFFLATIONS

These are the finely divided powders meant for introduction into the body cavities such as ears, nose, tooth sockets and vagina with the help of an apparatus known as insufflator. This divides the powder into a stream of finely divided particles to the site of application. The major difficulty in using this apparatus is that (i) it is difficult to obtain a measured quantity of drug to get a uniform dose; (ii) it has a tendency to get blocked when the powders used are wet or the apparatus itself is wet. The introduction of newer pressure aerosols have eliminated these difficulties. This method has the advantage that a measured quantity of dose through metered valves is supplied and the product is also protected.

In insufflations the particle size must be very small and they should be absolutely free from irritant and sensitizing effects.

SNUFFS

Snuffs are the finely divided solid dosage form of medicament which are inhaled into the nostrils for their antiseptic, decongestion or bronchodialator action. Snuffs should be dispensed in flat metal boxes with hinged lid.

DENTIFRICES

Dentifrices are the substances which are generally used with the help of tooth brush for cleaning the surfaces of the teeth. They are available in the form of fine powders and pastes.

For the preparation of tooth powders the same general principles already described for mixing the powders are applied. It is important to obtain the cleansing action chiefly by the detergent properties of the powder rather than through the use of harmful abrasives. A mild degree of abrasion is desirable which may be obtained by using chiefly finely precipitated calcium carbonate, one or more of the dibasic calcium phosphate, calcium sulphate, magnesium carbonate, sodium bicarbonate and sodium chloride. They also contain flavours and soap. Tooth pastes contain liquids such as glycerin, sorbitol, water and alcohol. A thickening agent like starch, tragacanth and cellulose derivatives is also incorporated. The sweetening agent added may be sugar but non-carbohydrate sweetening agents are preferred. Saccharin is generally used for this purpose.

The use of strong abrasive substances is harmful because it may damage the tooth structure. Similarly the dentifrices used by the dentist for cleaning purposes should not be used daily, it may spoil the teeth.

Rx

Hard soap in fine powder	5	gm
Precipitated calcium carbonate	93.5	gm
Saccharin sodium	0.3	gm
Clove oil	0.5	ml
Sod. lauryl sulphate	0.7	gm

Make a tooth powder.

Marketed Medicated Tooth Powders

1. Clinso-Dent (ICPA Health Products Pvt. Ltd., Ankleshwar - 393002).
2. Fixon flavoured denture (ICPA Health Products Pvt. Ltd., Ankleshwar - 393002).
3. Steradent denture cleansing powder (Reckitt & Colman, Calcutta - 700071).

Marketed Medicated Tooth Pastes

1. Emoform (Dentifrices, Trithala - 679534).

   Contains :

   Formalin in a pleasantly flavoured base.
2. Desent tooth paste (Indoco Remedies Ltd., Bombay - 400093).

   Contains :

   Stronium chloride 10% in a dentifrice base.
3. Mentadent G (Hindustan Lever Ltd., Bombay - 400020).
4. Senolin (Warren Pharmaceutical Pvt. Ltd., Bombay - 400058).
5. Sensoform (Warren Pharmaceutical Pvt. Ltd., Bombay - 400058).

CACHETS

Cachets are the solid unit dosage form of medicament in which the drug is enclosed in a tasteless sheet made by pouring a mixture of rice flour and water between two hot, polished, revolving cylinders. The water evaporates and a sheet of wafer is formed known as cachets. Cachets are also known as wafer capsules or capsula amylacea. These are used to enclose nauseous or disagreeable powders and can hold 0.2 to 1.5 gm of powder. Sodium aminosalicylate which is given in a dose of 12 gm daily in the treatment of tuberculosis is commonly prescribed in cachets.

Cachets are hard to swallow as such therefore before administration a cachet should be dipped in water for a few seconds and then placed on the tongue and swallowed with a draught of water. In this way the outer shell of the cachet is softened but the enclosed powder will remain intact. After swallowing, the cachet will disintegrate and the powder will be released.

Advantages

1. They are easy to prepare because no complicated machinery is required (as compared to tablets).
2. Drugs can be extemporaneously and quickly dispensed in cachets.
3. Comparatively large doses of drugs can be dispensed because once they have been softened by dipping in water, even large sizes can be swallowed easily (compared to large size hard capsules).
4. They disintegrate quickly in the stomach.

Disadvantages

1. They are easily damaged.
2. They do no protect the enclosed drugs from light and moisture.
3. They require moistening before swallowing.
4. They cover more space than the corresponding sizes of capsules or tablets.
5. The contents of cachets cannot be greatly compressed because of the fragile nature of the shells.
6. They cannot be filled by large-scale machinery.

Due to these disadvantages cachets are not very commonly used as that of capsules and tablets.

Types of Cachets

There are two types of cachets : (a) wet seal cachets which are sealed by moistening the edges with water; and (b) dry seal cachets which do not require any moisture for sealing.

(a) Wet Seal Cachets

A wet seal cachet is made up of two similar convex halves having flat edges. The weighed amount of powder is placed in one half, the edges of the other half are moistened with water and placed exactly over the first half containing the powder. The flat edges of both the halves are pressed together so that a perfect seal is made and the powder is completely enclosed.

Wet Seal Cachet Machine

This machine consists of three thin metal plates joined by hinges so that they may be opened or superposed as and when desired. The halves of the cachet in which the powder is to be filled are placed in the central plate where they fit loosely. The second plate having the corresponding holes like that of first plate is then superposed on the central plate. The object of this plate is to protect the edges of cachets while they are being filled. The powder is filled in the halves placed in first plate, by means of funnels supplied with the machine. The powder so filled is then pressed down with a small plunger or metal thimble also supplied with the machine.

After filling the lower halves, the second plate is folded back to its original position. The other halves of the cachets are then placed in the corresponding holes of the third plate. The edges of these halves are then moistened with water from a roller attached with the machine. This plate is turned over the central plate in such a way that the edges of two halves completely cover each other and little pressure is applied so as to join the two halves. The upper plate is then lifted upward which will bring the complete cachets with it. The finished cachets are gently removed from upper plate and securely packed in cardboard or tin boxes. Cachets should

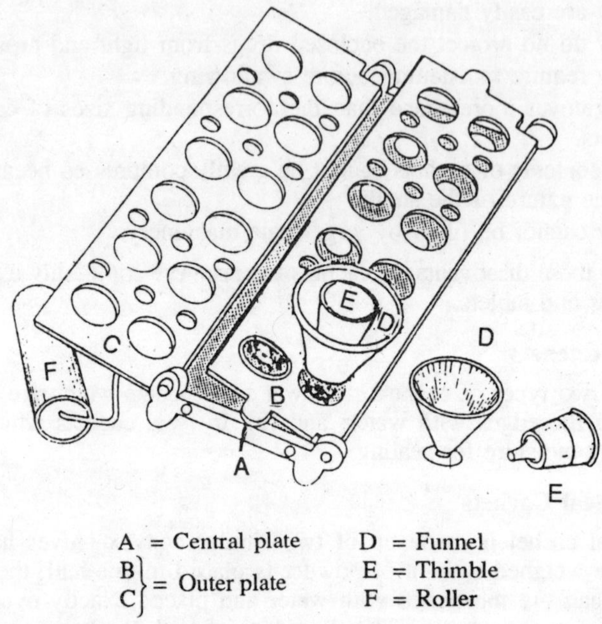

Fig. 4.1 Cachet machine.

be labelled with directions for administration, e.g., "Immerse in water for a few seconds and then swallow with a draught of water.".

(b) Dry Seal Cachets

Dry seal cachets consists of two halves, the upper half and the lower half, the former is little larger in diameter. The powder is filled in lower half and upper half is fitted over it like a lid on a box. The backs of upper as well as lower halves have small projections which are used to fix the cachet in the holes of the machine. The lower halves are fitted into the lower plate of the machine and powder filled therein. The upper halves are fitted in the upper plate by means of projections which will not allow

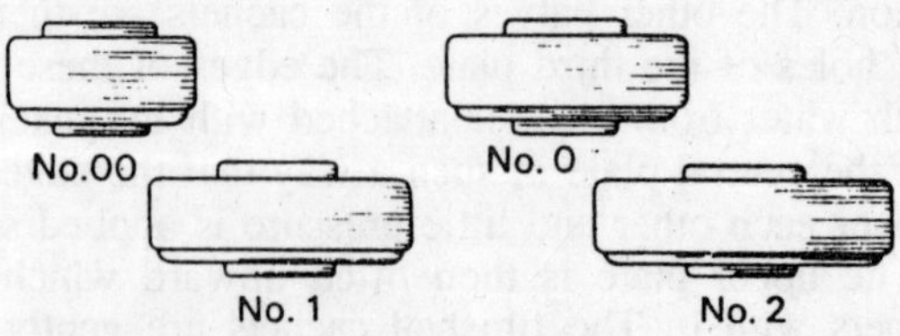

Fig. 4.2 Dry seal cachets.

the cachets to fall when the plate is removed. The upper plate is pressed down on the lower plate forcing the upper halves or lids to fit exactly over the lower halves. The filled cachets are removed and packed in boxes.

The dry seal cachets have advantages that there are no chances of escaping the powder and can be prepared more quickly and are more hygienic.

Dispensing

The catchets are dispensed in boxes or tins in which they are packed on their edges or lying flat. If necessary the compartments may be filled with cotton wool. Catchets should be labelled with directions for its use : "Immerse in water for a few seconds and then swallow with a draught of water.".

MOLDED TABLETS

1. Hypodermic tablets
2. Dispensing tablets.

Molded Tablets or Tablet Triturates "TT"

Molded tablets are small disk-shaped tablets which are prepared by forcing the soft mass into the cavities of the mold. Generally potent medicaments and highly toxic drugs in small doses are used for preparing the molded tablets. The potent medicament is diluted with a diluent like lactose, dextrose, sucrose, or a mixture of lactose and sucrose. The mixed powders are moistened with a suitable dilution of alcohol (generally 50% alcohol is used) and mixed thoroughly so as to get a soft mass. The soft mass so prepared is pressed into the perforations of the mold with a spatula. The excess of the mass is removed by applying pressure over the spatula. This perforated plate having exactly the same number of projecting pegs as that

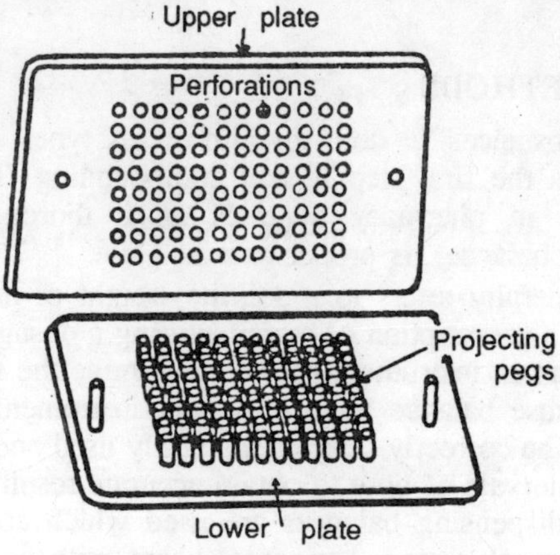

Fig. 4.3 Tablet triturate mold.

of perforations and these projecting pegs completely fit into the holes. A little pressure is applied over the top plate which will force the plate move downward, leaving the molded tablets on the projecting pegs. The ejected tablets are spread in single layers on clean surface and dried either by keeping in warm place or hot air oven.

Now a days tablet triturates may also be prepared on automatic tablet triturate machines including tablet making machines. A tablet triturate machine can prepare 2500 tablet triturates per minute.

Hypodermic Tablets

Hypodermic tablets are soft, readily soluble tablets which are made in a tablet triturate mold. They are used for preparing solutions to be injected, therefore in selecting the materials used for preparing the hypodermic tablets care must be taken that they should be completely and readily soluble and no insoluble particle should be present. They should be free from bacterial contamination and proper precautions should be taken during molding regarding contamination and cleanliness.

Since the solutions prepared from hypodermic tablets are rarely sterile and a number of sterile parenteral solutions are now available therefore the use of hypodermic tablets for preparing solutions for injections is being discouraged.

Dispensing Tablets

These tablets are prepared for providing an accurate and convenient quantity of a potent drug that can be incorporated readily in compounding other dosage forms, e.g., liquids, powders or capsules, thus eliminating the necessity of weighing small quantities of potent substances. These tablets are solely designed to provide a convenient quantity for extemporaneous compounding and should never be dispensed for administration as a dosage form because sometimes they contain very potent drugs which may prove fatal.

WEIGHING METHODS

Weighing of substances is done in almost all types of pharmaceutical operations and is the first step in any compounding. The success of all these operations in pharmacy depends on a thorough knowledge of principles of the balance, its proper care and use.

Weighing generally refers to a definite weight of material to be used in compounding a prescription or manufacturing a dosage form. A balance may be defined as an instrument used to determine the relative weights of substances. Because balance is an important instrument for a pharmacist therefore it must be correctly selected, carefully used and properly checked after specified intervals of time to obtain accurate results. For prescription work generally dispensing balances are used which consist of a simple, light but rigid, equal armed, horizontal beam with central and terminal knife edges of steel which work in agate or steel bearing. Two pans are suspended from the terminal knife edges. When the load is placed in the pans the beam turns about the central fulcrum and deflection from the horizontal is indicated by movement of a pointer fixed below the centre of the beam. For weighing the materials the following techniques should be followed :

1. Place the balance in a well lighted location and in a convenient position for use. The area should be free from dust and there should be no corrosive vapours present nor high humidity or vibrations due to air currents.
2. Adjust the level of the balance.
3. Clean the pans with a clean cloth.
4. Place equal size powder papers (preferably wax paper) on each pan of the balance. They will prevent inaccuracy due to powder adhering to the pan and also to protect the pans from corrosion.
5. Place the required weights on the right hand pan with the help of forceps. The use of forceps will prevent inaccuracies in weighing due to sweat and grease from hands. Some of the writers suggest that the weights should be placed in the left hand pan and material to be weighed in the right hand pan. The left hand pan is less convenient because the pillar of the balance comes in the way but most of the workers prefer to use right hand pan for keeping the weights and left hand pan for keeping the material to be weighed.
6. Close the drawer of the balance which will prevent spillage of the powder on the weights lying in the drawer.
7. Remove the bottle of medicament from the shelf and check its label for the correct ingredient mentioned in the prescription.
8. Place the material to be weighed in the left hand pan. While taking out the material from the bottle hold the bottle in the left hand with the label upper most so that it is visible during weighing. Gently release the pan arrest to determine whether too much or too little material was added.
9. Remove or add the material, always using a spatula, after arresting the pan each time whenever transfer of material is made.
10. When the weights on the two pans will be equal the release of the pan arrest will show a zero rest point and the weighing is complete.
11. When the weighing is complete put the balance beam again in the fixed position.
12. Transfer the weighed material from the weighing paper to the compounding device and discard the weighing paper. Each time a new weighing paper should be used and readjusting of the balance equilibrium to a zero rest point must be done.
13. Return the weights to the drawer with forceps and carefully clean the balance pans and spatula.

14. Close the stock bottles and again check its labels. Return the bottles to the shelf. Preferably only one bottle should be removed from the shelf at a time for weighing and the same should be replaced immediately after the material is weighed. Then the next bottle should be removed and material weighed. This will avoid the mistakes which may be made if several bottles are kept on the bench together.

Possible Errors in Weighing

Errors in weighing may occur due to one or more of the following reasons :

1. If the balance is not leveled.
2. If the rest point of the balance is not correct.
3. If the two pans of the balance are of unequal weight.
4. If the pans are rough.
5. If the material is weighed directly on the pans.
6. If the weight of the material is taken while the pans are still oscillating.
7. If the weights are removed with fingers and not with forceps.
8. If the volatile substances are weighed in an open vessel.

Minimum Weighable Amounts

The maximum allowable error in weighing on a prescription balance is not more than ±5%. This value is significant only in very small weighings and efforts should be made to get a higher degree of accuracy. This figure indicates that of 100 mg of any substance is to be supplied then it must not be less than 95 mg and not more than 105 mg. But efforts should be made to weigh as near to 100 mg as possible. Since Smith's results showed that only 2 gr or more weighings were within ±5% errors therefore it is advisable not to weigh less than 100 mg (or 2 gr) on a prescription balance otherwise accurate weights will not be obtained. In any case amounts less than 50 mg (1 gr) should not be weighed on dispensing balance specially reserved for weighing quantities less than 100 mg or on general chemical balances.

Procedure for weighing below the minimum weighable amounts, geometrical dilutions :

The practice of dispensing powders in very small doses is obsolete but still some practitioners write prescriptions of powders in very small doses. Therefore following procedures should be followed for dispensing quantities below the minimum weighable amounts :

1. Very small quantities of materials may be weighed on a high grade analytical balance but the cost of such a balance might be prohibitive because the number of prescriptions requiring its use may be few. Therefore this method is not commonly used.

2. Prefabricated dosage forms such as tablet triturates, dispensing tablets and hypodermic tablets of the same drug may be used. Though this method is very convenient but may introduce an error.
3. The use of liquid and solid dilutions is the most suitable and convenient means of dispensing the small amounts of drugs accurately. In this method a minimum weighable quantity of the drug is weighed on a dispensing balance which is then mixed with a solid diluent such as lactose (for solid dosage forms) or water or any other solvent (for liquid dosage forms). Lactose is selected as diluent because it is white, sweet in taste, easily available, cheap and compatible with majority of the drugs.

While preparing triturations and dilutions the following limiting factors must be kept in mind :

1. The quantity of active medicament to be diluted must not be less than the minimum weighable amount.
2. The final dilutions prepared must represent the desired amount of the drug in the minimum weighable amounts.

When a very small quantity of drug is to be dispensed the best method is to prepare triturations and dilutions by using lactose as diluent. The general procedure is as follows :

Weigh 100 mg (minimum weighable amount) of the drug. Mix it gradually or by means of geometrical dilutions with the required quantity of lactose. Then weigh a portion of the mixed material which will contain the desired weight of the potent drug.

TRITURATIONS

The term trituration is applied to a mixture or dilution of a potent substance with an inert substance. Small quantities of finely powdered solids may be mixed on a sheet of white paper by means of bone spatula or powder knife. If the quantities are large to be conveniently mixed on paper sheet then pestle and mortar should be used. The invariable rule is to add a small amount of the substance present in greater amount to whole of the substance present in lesser amount (generally potent substance) and mix thoroughly. The remaining amount of the substance present in larger amount is then incorporated gradually in small quantities at first which are subsequently increased until whole of it has been added. This method of mixing is known as geometrical dilutions which may be explained that when 100 mg of any potent drug is to be mixed with 900 mg of lactose the best method is to take out 100 mg of lactose from bulk and mix it with 100 mg of drug. Total of this mixture will be 100 + 100 = 200 mg. Again take out 200 mg of lactose and mix it with 200 mg of first mixture, total of this mixture will be 200 + 200 = 400 mg. In the next step again take out 400 mg of lactose and mix it intimately with the second mixed material, total of this will be 400 + 400 = 800 mg. To this 800 mg add whole of the remaining lactose and mix thoroughly so as to get a uniform powder.

By geometrical dilution method very small quantities of drugs can be mixed intimately with large quantities of diluents and a uniform powder will be obtained whereas it is impossible to get intimate dispersion of one powder in another by mixing the two substances all at once.

In the case of costly drugs it becomes necessary to give a thought to cost factor of the drug but under no circumstances the compounding accuracy should be compromised with economy.

Proper care and usage of dispensing balance

It is the general tendency of the pharmacists that they do not take proper care of balance while using it, cleaning it or protecting it while it is not used. As balance is the most important instrument for a pharmacist and in almost all kinds of prescriptions the need arises to use a balance at one stage or the other therefore proper care of a balance must be taken while using, cleaning and storing it. In this regard following points must be taken care of :

1. It should be kept in a place where there is no dust, dampness, corrosive vapours and vibrations.
2. The balance should be kept on a leveled surface which should be hard like bench or table.
3. The analytical balances are protected by enclosing in glass cases provided with doors in the front and in the sides. While weighing any substance these doors must be kept closed.
4. Always clean the pans and surfaces of the balance with a clean dry duster before its use as well as after its use.
5. While using a balance neither the weights nor the substance that is to be weighed should be kept on the pans while the beam is free to oscillate.
6. Greasy and waxy substances should be weighed on a carefully counterbalanced sheet of wax paper. Preferably all substances should be weighed by placing counterbalanced wax paper in each of the pans.
7. Substances which act as metals such as iodine, corrosive sublimate, etc., should not be weighed directly on the pans but on counter-balanced watch glass.
8. Any agent spilled on the balance during use should be wiped off immediately with a soft brush or cloth.
9. While weighing, the drawer of the balance should be closed.
10. Weights should be transferred with forceps.
11. All materials should be transferred with spatula.

12. While cleaning the balance great care should be taken so that the delicate mechanism of the balance is not disturbed. Soft cloth or brush should be used for cleaning the balance.
13. When the balance is not in use, it must be cleaned and covered with the balance cover.

If due consideration is given to the above mentioned points in handling and using the balance it may give accurate weighings, correct results and last for a long time.

Revision Questions

I. Very short answer type question

Define the following :

(a) Powders
(b) Compound powders
(c) Dusting powders
(d) Potent powders
(e) Effervescent powders
(f) Bulk powders
(g) Tablet triturates
(h) Catchets
(i) Vegetable powders

II. Fill in the blanks

(a) Powders, which absorb moisture from the atmosphere, are known as ...... powders.
(b) When two or more than two powders are mixed together, they are known as ...... powders?
(c) Dusting powders are passed through sieve no 120 to remove ...... particles.
(d) Catchets are also known as ....
(e) The main ingredients of effervescent granules are 1. ...... 2. ...... 3. ....

III. Short answer type questions

1. Define powders and classify them
2. Explain advantages and disadvantages of powders
3. Describe a procedure by which liquids can be dispensed in powders
4. Describe in brief about geometrical dilution.
5. Discuss about proper care and usage of dispensing balance.

IV. Long answer type questions

1. What are powders? Explain advantages and disadvantages of powders. Classify powders and explain how will you dispense compound powder in divided doses.
2. How will you dispense the following in powders?
   (a) Vegetable powders
   (b) Hygroscopic and deliquescent substances
   (c) Eutectic substances
   (d) Liquids
   (e) Explosive substances
   (f) Potent drugs.
3. What are effervescent granules? Discuss methods of preparation of effervescent granules.
4. Define cachets. Discuss advantages and disadvantages of cachets. Describe method of preparation of cachets.
5. What are cachets? Discuss different types of cachets and their method of preparation.
6. Discuss what are tablet triturates their types and methods of preparation?
7. Write short notes on the following.
   (a) Effervescent granules
   (b) Granular powders
   (c) Eutectic substances.
   (d) Dusting powders
   (e) Bulk powders
   (f) Potent powders
   (g) Dentifrices
   (h) Insufflations
   (i) Cachets
   (j) Tablet triturates
8. How will you dispense following in powders?
   (a) Hygroscopic and deliquescent substances
   (b) Eutectic substances
   (c) Vegetable powders
   (d) Liquids
   (e) Explosive substances
   (f) Potent drugs.
9. Differentiate between the followings :
   (a) Simple powders and compound powders
   (b) Bulk powders for internal use and dusting powders.
   (c) Tablet triturates and cachets.
   (d) Effervescent powders and effervescent granules.

10. Name at least three marketed preparations of the following pharmaceuticals :
    (a) Dry syrups
    (b) Effervescent powders
    (c) Dusting powders
    (d) Medicated tooth pastes
    (e) Rehydration powders
11. Discuss possible errors in weighing and discuss proper care and usage of dispensing balance.

Answers

(a) Hygroscopic and deliquescent
(b) Compound
(c) Gritty particles
(d) Wafer capsules
(e) Citric acid, tartaric acid, sodium bicarbonate.

5

Monophasic Liquid Dosage Forms

A solution is a clear, homogeneous mixture that is prepared by dissolving a solid, liquid or gas in another liquid. The component of a solution present in large amount is known as solvent and the component present in lesser amount is known as solute. A solution is homogeneous because the solute is in a molecular or ionic state of subdivision, therefore, a true solution is a one phase system. Solutions may be used internally or applied externally whereas mixtures are meant for oral administration. Mixtures are mainly prescribed for acute conditions such as cough, indigestion, diarrhoea, constipation and rheumatism. They are prepared extemporaneously and supplied only for a few days treatment because if they are stored for more than a few weeks even under normal conditions they may deteriorate.

Advantages

1. They are homogeneous, therefore the medicament is uniformly distributed throughout the liquid.
2. The doses can be easily adjusted according to the need of the patient.
3. They can be easily measured with the household measures.
4. They are more quickly effective than tablets or capsules because they are already in the solution form and absorption starts quickly.
5. Some drugs like potassium iodide and bromide leads to gastric pain if taken in the tablet or capsule form but this pain may be reduced when these drugs are administered in the solution form because of dilution factor.
6. They can be easily coloured, flavoured or sweetened.
7. Children or patients who cannot swallow tablets or capsules can easily ingest solutions.
8. There are certain drugs which can only be administered in liquid dosage form, e.g., castor oil and liquid paraffin, etc.

Disadvantages

1. They are difficult to carry and there are chances of breakage of container with the complete loss of contents.
2. In some medicaments their unpleasant taste and flavour is difficult to mask.
3. They are less stable as compared to solid dosage forms because deterioration is faster in solutions.

SOLUBILITY

When an excess of a solid is brought in contact with the solvent and the solid is allowed to dissolve in the solvent, after some time a stage is reached when an equilibrium is established between the solute and the solvent and no more solute dissolves, the resulting solution is said to be saturated at that temperature and the extent to which the solute dissolves is known as its solubility. A solution is said to be supersaturated when it contains a larger amount of the solute than is necessary to form a saturated solution at a particular temperature. These supersaturated solutions create formulation problems because they deposit the excess of substance upon standing and lead to undesirable results. Temperature of 20°C is considered the optimum temperature for the preparation of stable saturated solutions because this is the room temperature at which the medicines are supposed to be kept and used.

Most substances whether solid, liquid or gas can be dissolved in some liquid but none is soluble in all liquids, some of them may be poorly soluble, slightly soluble, highly soluble or even may be insoluble. Water is always considered the most suitable vehicle for the preparation of liquid formulations but a large number of modern drugs are insoluble in it. Hence the solubility of most of these compounds can be increased by one or more of the following methods :

1. Solubilization
2. Co-solvency
3. Complexation
4. Hydrotrophy
5. Chemical modification of the drug
6. pH adjustments.

(a) Solubilization

Solubilization is the process in which the water insoluble substances are dissolved in aqueous solutions in the presence of surfactants. The mechanism for this phenomenon is that the surface active agents when added to the solution to be formed tend to aggregate in groups of 100-150 molecules known as micelles. This phenomenon occurs at a certain concentration of surfactant which is known as critical micelle concentration or CMC. Solubilization occurs either by dissolving the solute in the micelle or the solute is adsorbed on to the micelle. Thus the solubilization starts at critical micelle concentration and generally increases with increase in the concentration of micelles.

The solutions so formed are thermodynamically stable. Hence the phenomenon of solubilization is widely used in the development of pharmaceutical formulations. Many water-insoluble drugs are formulated as clear, aqueous solutions by the process of miceller solubilization. A number of drugs can be solubilized in a variety of solvents by using different surface active agents. The examples of drugs which can be solubilized are : fat soluble vitamins A, D, E & K; antibiotics like chloramphenicol, griseofulvin and amphotericin B; analgesics like aspirin, acetanilide and phenacetin, etc. Many alkaloids and glycosides are also solubilized in this way.

(b) Co-Solvency

The solubility of poorly soluble drugs in water can be increased by mixing it with some water miscible solvent in which the drug is readily soluble. This phenomenon is known as co-solvency and the solvents used in combination to increase the solubility of the solute are known as co-solvents. Most of the solvent mixtures consist of water, alcohol, glycerin, propylene glycol and syrups.

(c) Complexation

Insoluble substances often react with a soluble ingredient to form a complex which is readily soluble in water. A very common example of this type is the formation of tri-iodide complex when iodine and potassium iodide are mixed together. Iodine is insoluble in water whereas the tri-iodide complex so formed is readily soluble in water. The solubility of caffeine is 1 : 50 whereas the solubility of caffeine and sodium benzoate is 1 : 1.2 in water. When the solubility is increased by complexation, one has to make sure that the complex formed is reversible, dissociates easily and releases the active ingredients readily otherwise the active ingredient becomes therapeutically ineffective.

(d) Hydrotrophy

The term hydrotrophy refers to the increase in solubility of insoluble or slightly soluble drugs in water by the addition of additives, which are not surface active agents. The exact mechanism by which this effect occurs is not clear. The mechanism might be a solubilization, complexation, co-solvency or a combination of several factors. The phenomenon has very little use in pharmaceutical systems.

(e) Chemical Modification of the Drug

Many drugs which are poorly soluble in water can be chemically converted into their derivatives which are appreciably soluble in water. For example, alkaloids are poorly soluble in water whereas alkaloidal salts are freely soluble in water. Similarly many other drugs like corticosteroids, etc., can be converted into water soluble derivatives. This approach is highly successful in certain types of drugs but has several practical limitations.

(f) pH Adjustments

The solubilities of chemotherapeutic agents which are weak acids or weak bases can be markedly influenced by variations in pH. However, this is not always the best course of action. Before adjusting the pH of any preparation, numerous other implications must also be taken into consideration which may markedly affect the stability of the preparation.

Other Formulation Problems

It is not sufficient to formulate a liquid dosage form that has the desired concentrations of the active ingredients, pH, colour, taste and flavour but should also be chemically and physically stable. The chemical stability of the active ingredients of the formulation are of primary importance and the formulation should be designed to minimize hydrolysis, oxidation, reduction, polymerization or any other chemical change of the active ingredients. Instability also includes variation in colour, flavours, cloudiness or precipitation, bacterial growth, viscosity decrease, etc. Caking of suspensions or cracking of emulsions also leads to instability of preparations. Because of these problems it is difficult to prepare liquid dosage forms with an extended stability, therefore many drugs are prepared in the form of powders which are required to be dissolved in a suitable vehicle immediately before its use.

Liquid preparations which are to be administered into the eyes or meant for parenteral administration must be sterile and they should be isotonic with the lacrymal secretions or blood serum as the case may be. Oral preparations should be elegant in appearance, colour, flavour, taste, etc. They should possess the desirable viscosity as regards to pourability, stability and effectiveness.

LIQUID FORMULATIONS FOR INTERNAL USE

Mixtures

A mixture is a liquid preparation intended for oral administration in which drug or drugs are dissolved, suspended or dispersed in a suitable vehicle and generally several doses are contained in a bottle. When only one dose is dispensed it is known as draught.

Mixtures differ from solutions that the mixtures may be homogeneous or heterogeneous and are for oral administration whereas solutions are homogeneous and are for external or internal use. Mixtures are extemporaneously prepared and they are supplied in such doses that whole of the mixture is used up within a few days. If need arises then fresh mixture is prepared.

Advantages of Mixtures

1. They are more quickly effective than solid dosage forms which require previous disintegration in the body before absorption can take place.
2. Certain substances can only be given in liquid form because they are inconvenient to administer in any other form due to their liquid nature and large dose, e.g., castor oil, liquid paraffin, aromatic waters, etc.
3. Certain substances like potassium iodide and potassium bromide may cause pain in the stomach if given in the solid form as a powder or a tablet.
4. Certain substances are useful when they are administered in a suspension form, e.g., light kaolin and bismuth salts, because in suspension form they afford large surface area for the absorption of toxic substances in the gut.
5. Mixtures are easy to administer and economical as compared to other oral preparations.

Disadvantages

1. They are comparatively less stable than solid dosage forms.
2. Incompatibility is more in liquid preparations as compared to solid ones.
3. They are more bulky and difficult to carry.

Classification

Mixtures may be classified as follows :

1. Simple mixtures
2. Mixtures containing diffusible solids
3. Mixtures containing indiffusible solids
4. Mixtures containing precipitate forming liquids
5. Mixtures containing slightly soluble liquids
6. Miscellaneous mixtures.

Simple Mixtures

A simple mixture is one which contains only soluble ingredients, e.g., carminative mixture, diaphoretic mixture, cough expectorant, etc.

Method of Dispensing

(a) Dissolve the solid substances in ¾th of the vehicle. The reasons for this is that (i) the volume occupied by the other ingredients rarely exceeds the remaining ¼th, but if this volume exceeds, the ¾th quantity of vehicle used must be reduced; (ii) solution formation is hastened by using as much of the solvent as convenient.

(b) Examine the solution critically by holding the container against light. If foreign particles are visible pass the solution through cotton wool, further pour little more vehicle over cotton wool so that the solution therein is removed.
(c) Add any liquid ingredients. Volatile liquids are added at the end just before adjusting the final volume with vehicle.
(d) Add more of vehicle to produce the final volume.
(e) Transfer the mixture to a bottle, cork, and thoroughly polish the bottle to remove finger prints. Attach the label, wrap the bottle and dispense.

Mixtures containing diffusible solids and indiffusible solids are discussed under suspensions.

Marketed Mixtures/Liquid Preparations

1. Carminative mixture (Zandu Pharmaceutical Works Ltd., Bombay - 400025).

   Each contains :

   Sodium bicarbonate, Spt. ammonia aromatic, Tr. gentian comp., Tr. card. comp., Spt. chloroform, Tr. zingiberis.

2. Gelusil liquid (Warner-Hindustan Division, Bombay - 400072).

   Each 5 ml contains :

Magnesium trisilicate	625 mg
Dried aluminium hydroxide gel	312 mg

3. Kaolin mixture (Arora Pharmaceuticals Pvt. Ltd., New Delhi - 110035).

   Each 15 ml contains :

Light kaolin	2	mg
Light mag. carbonate	0.6	gm
Sodium bicarbonate	0.6	gm
Peppermint water	15	ml

4. Kloratum liquid (Klar Sehen Pvt. Ltd., Calcutta - 700026).

   Each 5 ml contains :

Pot. chloride	500 mg

5. Lederplex liquid (Cyanamid India Ltd., Lederle Division, Bombay - 400025).

Marketed Solutions

1. Acriflavine solution (Agrawal Pharmaceuticals, Delhi - 110092).

   Each ml contains :

Acriflavine	0.1%

2. Cetrimide HC 0.5% liquid (I.C.I. India Ltd., Madras - 600008).

   Contains :

Cetrimide	0.5% w/w
Chlorhexidine HCl	0.1% w/w

3. Dettol antiseptic liquid (Reckitt & Colman of India Ltd., Calcutta 700071).

   Contains :

Chloroxylenol	4.8%	w/v
Terpineol	9%	v/v
Absolute alcohol	13.1%	v/v

4. Merbromin solution (Agrawal Pharmaceuticals, Delhi - 110092).

   Contains :

   Merbromin 2%

5. Savlon hospital concentrate liquid (I.C.I. India Ltd., Madras 600008).

   Contains :

Chlorhexidine gluconate	7.5%	v/v
Cetrimide	15%	w/w

SYRUPS

Syrups are the sweet, viscous, concentrated aqueous solutions of sucrose or other sugars in water or any other suitable aqueous vehicle. When purified water alone is used in making the solution of sucrose the preparation is known as syrup or simple syrup. When the preparation contains some medicinal substance it is known as medicated syrup. When the syrup does not contain any medicament but contains various aromatic or pleasantly flavoured substances are known as flavouring syrups. They are used for masking the disagreeable taste of bitter or saline drugs. They are also used as vehicles or flavours for extemporaneous preparations.

In addition to sucrose, certain other polyols, such as glycerin, sorbitol or other polyhydric alcohols may be added in small amounts to retard crystallization of sucrose or to increase the solubility of other added ingredients.

In the manufacture of syrups the sucrose and purified water free from foreign substances should be selected and clean containers must be used to avoid contamination during preparation. Dilute solutions of sucrose support mold, yeast and other microbial growth whereas the growth of such microorganisms is usually retarded when the concentration of sucrose is 65% weight by weight or more but a saturated solution may lead to crystallization of sucrose.

Only small quantities of syrups should be prepared which can be used within a few months. If large quantities are to be prepared then they must be preserved well to prevent contamination. Syrups can be well preserved at a temperature not exceeding 25°C. In dilute solutions preservatives like glycerin, methyl paraben, benzoic acid and sodium benzoate may be added.

Now a days artificial syrups prepared from artificial sweetening agents are available in the market. They have the advantage over syrups prepared from sugars that they do not contain any carbohydrate therefore can be easily given to diabetic patients. Moreover they have lesser stability problems than sugar-based syrups.

Examples are syrup, orange syrup, tolu syrup, raspberry syrup, black currant syrup and wild cherry syrup.

Storage : Syrups should be stored in a well-closed container and at a temperature not exceeding 30°C.

Marketed Syrups

1. Benadryl syrup [Parke-Davis (India) Ltd., Bombay - 400025].

   Each 5 ml contains :

Diphenhydramine HCl	12.5 mg

2. Corex cough syrup (Pfizer Ltd., Bombay - 400021).

   Each 5 ml contains :

Chlorpheniramine maleate	4	mg
Codein phos.	10	mg
Ephedrine HCl	5	mg
Sod. citrate	150	mg
Menthol	0.1	mg

3. Crocin syrup (Duphar-Interfran Ltd., Bombay - 400018).

   Each 5 ml contains :

Paracetamol	125 mg

4. Metacin syrup (Themis Pharmaceuticals, Bombay - 400093).

   Each 5 ml contains :

Paracetamol	0.125 gm

5. Polybion syrup [E. Merck (India) Ltd., Bombay - 400018]. Multivitamin preparation.
6. Sudafed syrup [Burroughs Wellcome (India) Ltd., Bombay - 400023].
7. Ultragin syrup (Geoffrey Manners & Co. Ltd., Bombay - 400038).

   Each 5 ml contains :

Analgin	15.62 mg
Paracetamol	15.62 mg

8. Vi-Syneral syrup [U.S. Vitamin (India) Ltd., Bombay - 400018]. Multivitamin preparation.

ELIXIRS

Elixirs are clear, pleasantly flavoured, sweetened hydroalcoholic liquid preparations for oral administration. The main ingredients of elixirs are ethanol and water but glycerin, sorbitol, propylene glycol, flavouring agents, sugar and preservatives may be incorporated to the preparation. The elixirs may be medicated or non-medicated. The medicated elixirs usually contain very potent drugs such as antibiotics, antihistaminics and sedatives. The bitter and nauseous taste of certain drugs can be masked by adding flavouring and sweetening agents. The non-medicated elixirs are used as flavours and vehicles.

Examples are chloral elixir, chlorpheniramine elixir, paracetamol elixir, phenobarbitone elixir, piperazine citrate elixir.

Storage : Since elixirs contain alcohol and usually some volatile oils which deteriorate in the presence of air and light therefore they should be stored in tightly closed, light resistant containers and in a cool place.

Marketed Elixirs

1. Betonin (Vitamin B-Complex) elixir (Boots Pharmaceuticals Ltd., Bombay - 400038).
2. Cadiphylate elixir (Cadila Laboratories Ltd., Ahmedabad - 380050).

   Each 5 ml contains :

Theophylline ethanoate of piperazine	80	mg
Ephedrine HCl	12	mg
Glyceryl guaiacolate ether	50	mg
Phenobarbitone	4	mg
Alcohol	0.55	ml

3. Ephedrine compound elixir [Parke-Davis (India) Ltd., Bombay - 400025].

   Each 5 ml contains :

Ephedrine sulphate	22.80	mg
Caffeine	91.2	mg
Sod. salicylate	114.0	mg
Sod. iodide	60.8	mg
Ext. of belladonna green	14.25	mg
Alcohol	0.787	ml
Alcohol content	15%	v/v

4. Phosfomin tonic elixir (Sarabhai Chemicals, Vadodra - 390007).
5. Phosfomin iron tonic elixir (Sarabhai Chemicals, Vadodra - 390007).
6. Piperazine elixir [Burroughs Wellcome (India) Ltd., Bombay - 400023].
7. Rubraplex elixir (Sarabhai Chemicals, Vadodra - 390007).

LINCTUSES

LInctuses are sweet, viscous liquid preparations usually containing medicinal substances which have demulcent, sedative or expectorant properties. They are used for the treatment of cough. They produce soothening effect on the mucous membrane of the throat. To obtain the maximum effect they should be taken in small doses, sipped and swallowed slowly without the addition of water.

Examples are codeine linctus, noscapine linctus, simple linctus.

Marketed Linctuses

1. Coskin linctus (Warner-Hindustan Division, Bombay - 400072).

Each 5 ml contains :

Noscapine	15	mg
Glyceryl guaiacolate	100	mg
Chlorpheniramine maleate	2	mg
Spirit chloroform	0.4	ml
Menthol	1	mg
Alcohol content	8-10%	v/v

2. Coscopin linctus (Biological E. Ltd., Hyderabad - 500020).
3. Protussa cough linctus (Boots Pharmaceuticals Ltd., Bombay 400038).

Each 5 ml contains :

Noscapine	5	mg
Sod. citrate	125	mg
Ephedrine HCl	3	mg
Tinct. belladonna	0.125	ml
Tolu solution	0.133	ml

Marketed Expectorants

1. Avil expectorant (Hoechst India Ltd., Bombay - 400021).
2. Benadryl cough expectorant [Parke-Davis (India) Ltd., Bombay - 400025].
3. Broncare expectorant (Themis Pharmaceuticals, Bombay - 400093).
4. Novadin expectorant (Novus Pharmaceuticals, Bombay - 400093).
5. Piritone Glaxo expectorant (Glaxo India Ltd., Bombay - 400025).

Each 5 ml contains :

Chlorpheniramine maleate	2.5 mg
Amm. chloride	125.0 mg
Sod. citrate	55.0 mg

DROPS

These are liquid preparations meant for oral administration. Generally potent medicaments and vitamins are formulated as drops. Usually vitamin A and D concentrates in fish liver oil are presented as drops for administration to children. Since these drops contain potent medicaments, the dose must be measured precisely with droppers which are accurately graduated in fractions of a millilitre.

Marketed Drops

1. Abdec drops [Parke-Davis (India) Ltd., Bombay - 400025].
   Multivitamin drops.
2. Arovit drops (Roche Products Ltd., Bombay - 400034).

   Each ml contains :

Vit. A	150,000 I.U.
3. Crocin drops (Duphar-Interfran Ltd., Bombay - 400018).

   Each ml contains :

Paracetamol	150 mg
4. Digiplex drops (Rallis India Ltd., Bombay - 400001).

   Each ml contains :

Diastase	31.25 mg
Pepsin	10.0 mg
5. Incremin drops (Cyanamid India Ltd., Lederle Division, Bombay - 400025).

   Contains :

   Lysine and vitamins.
6. Metacin drops (Themis Pharmaceuticals, Bombay - 400093).
7. Sporidex drops (Ranbaxy Laboratories Ltd., New Delhi - 110019).

   Each ml contains :

Cephalexin	100 mg
8. Vi-Syneral vitamin drops [U.S. Vitamin (India) Ltd., Bombay - 400018].
   Multivitamin drops.
9. Toothache drops (Alpine Industries, New Delhi - 110028).

   Each contains :

Clove oil	5% w/v
Methyl salicylate	15% w/v
Camphor	1% w/v
Peppermint oil	6% w/v

DRAUGHTS

A draught is a liquid preparation taken as a single dose. If several doses are prescribed they are dispensed in separate containers but Ipecacuanha Emetic Draught is an exception in which several doses are prescribed in a multiple dose container.

Liquids for External Use

1. Liquids to be used in the mouth and other body cavities, e.g., gargles, mouth washes, throat paints, sprays, enemas, douches, nasal drops, inhalations, eye drops, eye lotions, ear drops, etc.
2. Liquids to be applied to the skin, e.g., liniments, lotions, etc.

1. Liquids to be Used in the Mouth and Other Body Cavities

Gargles

Gargles are aqueous solutions used for the treatment of an infection of the throat. Usually they are concentrated solutions and must be diluted with water before use. In using the gargles they are brought into intimate contact with the mucous membrane of the throat and are allowed to remain there for a few moments after which they are thrown out of the mouth.

Gargles should be dispensed in clear, fluted glass bottles closed with a plastic screw cap and labelled in such a way that it clearly distinguishes them from preparations meant for internal administration. If they are to be swallowed after use, they should be dispensed in bottles similar to the bottles used for mixtures. If the gargles are to be protected from light, they should be dispensed in light-resistant containers. Directions should be given on the label for diluting the gargles before use.

Examples are phenol gargles, potassium chlorate and phenol gargles.

Rx

Phenol glycerin	5 ml
Amaranth solution	1 ml
Water	up to 100 ml

Label : The gargles.
Sig : Dilute it with an equal volume of warm water before use.
Type : Gargles.

Procedure

Mix Amaranth solution (1% w/v in chloroform water) with small amount of water, add phenol glycerin (16% w/w phenol and 84% w/w glycerin) and mix. To this incorporate more of vehicle to produce the required volume. Transfer to a container, label and dispense. Secondary label "Not to be swallowed in large amounts" must be attached.

Uses

It is used as gargles for the treatment of pharynx and nasopharynx by forcing air from the lungs through the gargles which is held in the throat.

Phenol gargles should be diluted with an equal volume of warm water before use.

Mouth Washes

A mouth wash is an aqueous solution with a pleasant taste and odour used for rinsing, deodorant, refreshing or antiseptic action. It may contain alcohol, glycerin, sweetening agents, surface active agents, flavouring agents and colouring agents. Medicated mouth washes containing astringents, antibacterial agents, protein precipitants or other agents are also used but they must be used under the supervision of the dentist. A very simple preparation like compound sodium chloride mouth wash containing sodium chloride and sodium bicarbonate in peppermint water is commonly used. The medicated mouth washes should not be indiscriminately used by a normal person, the continuous use may prove harmful.

Mouth washes should be dispensed in clear fluted bottles. The container should be labelled with directions for diluting the mouth wash before use.

Rx

Sodium chloride	2 gm
Sodium bicarbonate	1 gm
Amaranth solution	2 ml
Peppermint water	up to 100 ml

Label : The mouth wash.

Directions :

1. Dilute it with an equal volume of warm water before use.
2. Rinse the mouth 3-4 times daily as required.

Type : Mouth wash.

Procedure

Dissolve the weighed quantities of sodium chloride and sodium bicarbonate in ¾th of the vehicle, add Amaranth solution and incorporate more of vehicle to produce the required volume. Transfer to a bottle, label and dispense. The secondary label "Not to be swallowed in large amounts" must be attached.

Uses

Compound sodium chloride mouth wash is a simple mouth wash which is used to cleanse and deodorise the buccal cavity. It is very refreshing particularly to the bed-ridden patients.

1. Sodium chloride makes the preparation isotonic.

2. Sodium bicarbonate can dissolve mucous therefore added to spray solutions and washes for the throat and nose.
3. Amaranth solution is used as a colouring agent.
4. Peppermint water is used to impart pleasant taste and odour to the preparation.

Marketed Mouth-washes and Gargles

1. Dettolin mouth wash and gargles (Reckitt & Colman of India Ltd., Calcutta - 700071).

   Contains :

Chloroxylenol	1.02%	w/v
Menthol	0.12%	w/v
Absolute alcohol	60.8%	v/v

   Amaranth as colour.

2. Garlin mouth-wash (Klar Sehen Pvt. Ltd., Calcutta - 700026).
3. Listrine liquid (Warner-Hindustan Division, Bombay - 400072).

   Contains :

Thymol	0.06%	w/v
Eucalyptol	0.09%	w/v
Methyl salicylate	0.06%	w/v
Menthol	0.04%	w/v
Benzoic acid	0.15%	w/v
Alcohol	25.27%	v/v

4. Thymoral mouth-wash (Rays Labs Pvt. Ltd., Calcutta - 700007).
5. Povidine mouth-wash (Stadmed Pvt. Ltd., Calcutta - 700071).

   Each contains :

   Povidone iodine 1% w/v

Throat Paints

Throat paints are viscous liquid preparations used for mouth and throat infections. In general the drugs used are antibiotics, sulphonamides, iodides, phenol and tannic acid. Glycerin is commonly used as a base because of its viscous nature and agreeable taste. Boroglycerin, phenol glycerin, tannic acid glycerin and compound iodine paint (Mandle's paint) are commonly used as throat paints. They are made viscous so that the drug should remain in contact with mucous membrane for sufficiently long time to produce its prolonged action.

Throat paints should be dispensed in airtight, coloured fluted bottles in order to distinguish them from preparations meant of internal use. Such containers should be fitted with glass stoppers or other suitable closures.

They should be stored in a cool place. The containers should be labelled with instructions "Not to be swallowed in large amounts".

Marketed Throat Paints

1. Candid mouth paint (Glenmark Pharmaceuticals Ltd., Bombay 400026).

   Each contains :

Clotrimazole	1%

2. Dentex gum paint (Dermocare Labs, Ahmedabad - 380001).

   Each contains :

Tannic acid	3%
Pot. iodide	2%
Iodine	0.5%
Thymol	0.2%
Menthol	0.2%
Camphor	0.2%

3. Gumtex gum paint (Arora Pharmaceuticals Pvt. Ltd., New Delhi - 110035).
4. Gum paint (Alpine Industries, New Delhi - 110028).
5. Mastic paint compound (Alpine Industries, New Delhi - 110028).
6. Megenta paint (Alpine Industries, New Delhi - 110028).
7. Paint of iodine compound (Mandle's paint) (Alpine Industries, New Delhi - 110028).
8. Paintex paint (Mendine Pharmaceuticals Pvt. Ltd., Calcutta - 700027).

   Each ml contains :

Clove oil	3%
Camphor	0.1%
Menthol	1%
Glycerin	5%
Iodine tincture	7%
Sol. ether	10%
Peppermint water conc.	15%
Alcohol	56%

Sprays

Throat sprays are the liquid preparations which are sprayed into the mouth for their laryngitis, pharyngitis and tonsillitis action. But mainly they are used to produce their action on the lungs for which they are sprayed with a special type of atomiser known as nebuliser. Adrenaline and atropine spray is used as a bronchodialator in asthma and hay fever.

Sprays should be dispensed in coloured fluted bottles labelled with the instructions :

(a) Not to be swallowed.
(b) The preparation should be stored in a cool place.
(c) A darkened solution must not be used.

Marketed Inhaler Sprays

1. Aerocort inhaler (Cipla Ltd., Bombay - 400008).
2. Asthalin inhaler (Cipla Ltd., Bombay - 400008).

   Each metered dose contains :
   Salbutamol sulphate 100 mcg
3. Autohaler inhaler (Cipla Ltd., Bombay - 400008).
4. Beclate inhaler (Cipla Ltd., Bombay - 400008).
5. Cromal-5 inhaler (Cipla Ltd., Bombay - 400008).

Enemas

Enemas are aqueous or oily solutions or suspensions intended for introduction into the rectum for their purgative, sedative, anthelmintic, anti-inflammatory or nutritive effects. They may also be used for x-ray examination of the lower bowel. Among the commonly used drugs in solution form which act as cleansing enemas include isotonic solution of sodium chloride, sodium bicarbonate 2%, sodium phosphate, magnesium sulphate, soap, glycerin and a combination of these substances. The other drugs used in the form of enemas include olive oil, arachis oil, chloral hydrate, paraldehyde, turpentine, alum, tannic acid and barium sulphate, etc.

Usually solutions in volume of 500 ml to 1000 ml, depending on the age and condition of the patient is introduced as enema. However the commercially availably concentrated enemas are introduced in small volumes of 100 to 200 ml. Large volume enemas should be warmed to body temperature before administration.

There are two type of enemas (i) evacuant enemas and (ii) retention enemas. Evacuant enemas may be given up to 2 litres whereas retention enemas do not normally exceed 100 ml in volume.

Disposable Enemas

Now a days enemas are available in disposable plastic bags. Such enemas include magnesium sulphate as evacuant enemas and prednisolone as retention enemas.

A typical example of evacuant enema :

Rx

Soft soap 25 gm
Purified water 500 ml

Label : The soap enema.
Sig : To be used as directed.
Type : Evacuant enema.

Procedure

Dissolve the soft soap in purified water. Transfer to a container, label and dispense. Attach the secondary label "For rectal use only" and dispense.

Uses

It is used as an evacuant enema.

Precaution

Large volume enemas should be warmed to body temperature before administration.

Marketed Medicated Enemas

1. Laxicon enema (Stadmed Pvt. Ltd., Calcutta - 700071).

   Each contains :

   Dioctyl sod. sulphosuccinate 0.25%

2. Practo-Clyss (Comteck Labs, Bombay - 400016).

   Each contains :

Sod. dihydrogen phosphate	16% w/w
Sod. phosphate I.P.	6% w/w
Purified water q.s.	

Douches

A douche is an aqueous solution meant for introduction into one of the body cavities either for medicinal treatment or for hygienic purposes. The word 'douche' is most commonly used for vaginal solutions and are generally called irrigations. Douches are also used to irrigate the eyes, ear or nasal cavities for cleaning or removing the foreign particles or discharges from these cavities.

Many douches are dispensed in the form of powders or tablets accompanied by directions for dissolving in a specified quantity of water, usually warm. They are also dispensed as concentrated solutions and the patient is required to dilute it accordingly before use.

Solutions commonly used as cleansing douche include water, sodium chloride (0.2% isotonic), boric acid 2%, sodium bicarbonate 2%. Medicated solutions include mercuric chloride 1 : 3000 to 1 : 10000, silver nitrate 1 : 1000, potassium permanganate 1 : 4000 or lactic acid 0.5 to 3%. Weak solutions of tannic acid, acetic acid or vinegar and alum are used as astringents. Potassium permanganate, peroxides or perborates may be used for their deodorizing effect.

The equipment used is known as douche can and consists of a metal or rubber container to hold the solution. To this is attached a rubber tube about 2 metre long fitted with a nozzle, which may be of glass or rubber. Generally 1 litre to 2 litre of solution is used as a douche.

Ear Drops

Ear drops are the liquid preparations in which the drugs are dissolved or suspended in a suitable vehicle like water, dilute alcohol, glycerin, propylene glycol or any other suitable solvent and are intended for instillation into the ear with a dropper. Generally propylene glycol, polyethylene glycol and glycerin are most commonly used vehicles. Water is disfavoured because it would face difficulty in mixing with the secretions of ear which are mainly fatty.

Ear drops are generally used for cleansing the ear, drying weeping surfaces, softening the wax and for treating the mild infections.

Ear drops are dispensed in coloured fluted bottles attached with a dropper or in suitable plastic containers. The containers should be labelled "For external use only.".

Rx

Sodium bicarbonate	5 gm
Glycerin	30 ml

Purified water, freshly boiled and cooled to 100 ml

Label : The ear drops.
Sig : 2-3 drops to be put into each ear as directed.
Type : Ear drops.

Procedure

Dissolve the sodium bicarbonate in about 60 ml of purified water, add the glycerin and sufficient purified water to produce the required volume, mix thoroughly. Transfer to a dropper bottle, label and dispense. Attach the secondary label "For external use only.".

Uses

Sodium bicarbonate ear drops are used to relieve itching in the ears.

Marketed Ear Drops

1. Chloramphenicol ear drops (Bombay Drug House Pvt. Ltd., Bombay - 400101).

   Each ml contains :

   Chloramphenicol 5%

2. Chloromycetin ear drops [Parke-Davis (India) Ltd., Bombay - 400025].

   Contains :

   Chloramphenicol 5%
   Benzocaine 1% in propylene glycol.

3. Dexacort-N eye/ear drops (Klar Sehen Pvt. Ltd., Calcutta - 700026).

Contains :

Neomycin sulphate	0.5%
Dexamethasone sod. phosphate	0.1%

4. O-Carb ear drops (Optho Remedies Pvt. Ltd., Allahabad - 211004).

Each ml contains :

Sod. bicarb.	34 mg
Phenol	0.0034 ml
Glycerin	0.34 ml

5. Ophthal eye/ear drops (Ophthal Remedies, Ahmedabad - 382455).

Each ml contains :

Boric acid	2%
Sod. borate	0.5%
Zinc sulphate	0.1%
Glycerin	2%

Inhalations

Inhalations are the liquid preparations containing volatile ingredients and are meant for local or systemic action on the nasal or respiratory tract. If the ingredients are volatile at room temperature, they may be placed on an absorbent pad and inhaled therefrom. In other cases, they may be added to warm water, but not boiling water and the vapours are inhaled for five to ten minutes.

Inhalations are used to relieve nasal congestion and inflammation of the respiratory tract. The common examples of inhalations are benzoin inhalation, menthol and eucalyptus inhalation, ephedrine inhalation and isoproterenol hydrochloride inhalation.

Another group of products known as inhalants are drugs or combinations of drugs that can be carried into the nasal passages by virtue of their high vapour pressure. The device by which the inhalants are administered is known as inhaler. The example of an inhalant is propyl-hexedrine inhalant (Benzedrex).

Rx

Menthol	2 gm
Eucalyptus oil	10 ml
Light magnesium carbonate	7 gm
Water	up to 100 ml

Make an inhalation.

Sig : One teaspoonful to be added to 500 ml hot water (about 65°C) and inhale the vapours.

Type : Aqueous inhalation.

Procedure

Dissolve the menthol in the eucalyptus oil, add the light magnesium carbonate and sufficient water to produce 100 ml. Stir well so as to get a homogenous product. Transfer to a container, label with directions "For external use only." and "Shake the bottle before use." and dispense.

Uses

It is used as an inhalation to remove congestion of the nostrils.

Light magnesium carbonate acts as a distributing agent to ensure uniform dispersion of the oil on shaking. Light magnesium carbonate does not interfere with free volatilisation of the oil when the inhalation is added to hot water for use.

Nasal Drops

Nasal drops are usually aqueous solutions intended for instillation into the nostrils by means of dropper. They are commonly used for their antiseptic, local analgesic or vasoconstrictor properties.

At one time, oily preparation containing liquid paraffin or vegetable oils as vehicle were used to prolong the action of the drug but now the use of oily vehicles in the preparation of nasal drops is discouraged because on prolonged use the oil retards the ciliary action of the nasal mucosa or drops of oil may enter the trachea and cause lipoid pneumonia. Therefore, an aqueous vehicle is considered advisable for nasal drops.

Whenever possible nasal drops should be made iso-osmotic with 0.9% sodium chloride, pH neutral and viscosity similar to nasal secretions which can be achieved by the addition of a thickening agent like 0.5% methyl cellulose. They should be dispensed in coloured fluted bottles attached with a dropper.

Marketed Nasal Drops

1. Betnisol-N nasal drops (Glaxo India Ltd., Bombay - 400025).

   Contains :

Betamethasone sodium phosphate	0.05%
Naphazoline nitrate	0.05%
Neomycin sulphate	0.5%

2. Decon nasal drops (Cadila Labs Ltd., Ahmedabad - 380050).

   Each ml contains :

Xylometazoline HCl	0.1%

3. Diconal nasal drops (Klar Sehen Pvt. Ltd., Calcutta - 700026).

   Contains :

Xylometazoline HCl	0.1%
Sodium chloride	0.9%
Glycerin	6.0%

4. Dristan nasal drops (Geoffrey Manners & Co. Ltd., Bombay 400038).
5. Fenox nasal drops (Boots Pharmaceuticals Ltd., Bombay - 400038).

   Contains :

Phenylephrine HCl	0.25%
Naphazoline nitrate	0.025%
Chlorbutol	0.35%

6. Otrivin drops (Hindustan Ciba-Geigy Ltd., Pharmaceuticals Division, Bombay - 400020).

   Contains :

Xylometazoline HCl	0.1%

Marketed Sprays

1. Fintal nasal spray (Rallis India Ltd., Bombay - 400001).

   Contains :

Sod. cromoglycate	2%	w/v
Benzalkonium chloride	0.01%	w/v

2. Healex spray (Rallis India Ltd., Bombay - 400001).

   Each ml contains :

Polyvinyl polymer	2.52%
Benzocaine	0.36%
Propellant	70.0%

3. Arjet spray (Cadila Chemicals Ltd., Ahmedabad - 380050).
4. Beclate nasal spray (Cipla Ltd., Bombay - 400008).

   Each metered inhalation supplies :

Beclomethasone dipropionate	50 mcg

5. Iodex pain spray (Eskayef Ltd., Bangalore - 560049).
6. Iodex burn spray (Eskayef Ltd., Bangalore - 560049).
7. Iodex antiseptic spray (Eskayef Ltd., Bangalore - 560049).

   Contains :

   Povidone iodine.

2. Liquids to be Applied to the Skin

Liniments

Liniments are liquid or semi-liquid preparations meant for external application to the skin. They contain substances possessing analgesic, rubefacient, smoothing or stimulating properties. Liniments are usually applied to the skin with friction and rubbing of the skin. They should not be applied to the broken skin. Liniments should be dispensed in coloured fluted bottles in order to distinguish from preparations meant for internal use.

The bottle should be labelled "For external use only.".

Examples are methyl salicylate liniment, turpentine liniment, white liniment.

Storage : Liniments should be stored in tightly closed containers. The containers must bear a label "For external use only." and "Shake the bottle well before use.".

Rx

Soft soap	3.75 gm
Camphor	2.50 gm
Turpentine oil	32.50 ml
Purified water	11.25 ml

Make : Liniment.

Direction : To be applied externally to the affected part with friction.

Type : Emulsion type liniment made with an alkali soap.

Procedure

Dissolve the camphor in turpentine oil in a dry container. Separately dissolve soft soap in small amount of purified water in a mortar. To this gradually add the camphor solution with thorough trituration after each addition until a thick creamy emulsion is formed. Add sufficient purified water to produce the required volume. Transfer the preparation to a bottle, label and dispense. Apply the secondary label "For external use only." and "Shake the bottle before use.".

Uses

It acts as an irritant, counter-irritant and rubefacient.

Liniment of turpentine is applied externally to the patients suffering from arthralgia (pain in the joints), myalgia (muscular pain), fibrositis (ligamental pain) and sprain.

1. Irritants are the agents or substances which do not directly destroy the tissues but cause inflammation in the area to which they are applied.
2. Rubefacients are the substances which produce congestion and redness of the area to which they are applied, producing the initial symptoms of irritation.
3. Counter-irritants are the agents or drugs which are applied locally to irritate the intact skin thus reducing or relieving another irritation or deep seated pain. They seem to work by producing an inflammation, thus increasing the flow of blood to the affected area. Physical counter-irritants include hot water bottles, radiant heat, short wave

diathermy and galvanic electric current. Chemical counterirritants include volatile substances like turpentine oil, camphor, menthol, thymol and methyl salicylate.

4. Since turpentine oil is a volatile oil which is not miscible with water, to make them miscible with each other soft soap has been used which acts as an emulsifying agent.
5. Turpentine oil is a volatile oil obtained by the distillation and rectification of turpentine which is an oleoresin obtained from various species of pinus.
6. Camphor is a volatile substance obtained from wood of cinnamomum camphora. It can be prepared synthetically. Externally it acts as a mild analgesic and rubefacient. It is used as a counter-irritant in the treatment of fibrositis and neuralgia.

Precautions

Liniments are not to be applied to the broken skin because they may produce excessive irritation of the skin.

Marketed Liniments

1. Turpentine liniment (Alpine Industries, New Delhi - 110028).

   Each contains :

Soft soap	90 gm
Camphor	50 gm
Turpentine oil	650 ml
Purified water to	1000 ml

2. Turpentine liniment (Agrawal Pharmaceuticals, Delhi - 110092).
3. Turpentine liniment (Arora Pharmaceuticals, Delhi - 110035).
4. Methyl salicylate liniment (Alpine Industries, New Delhi - 110028).

   Each contains :

Methyl salicylate	250 mg
Arachis oil to	1000 ml

Marketed Applications

1. Ascazol application (Indian National Drug Co. Pvt. Ltd., Calcutta - 700085).

   Contains :

Benzyl benzoate	25%

2. Benzyl benzoate application (Medo Chem Lab. Pvt. Ltd., Delhi - 110032).

   Each contains :

Benzyl benzoate	250 gm

Emulsifying wax	20 gm
Purified water to	1000 ml

3. Benzyl benzoate application (Agrawal Pharmaceuticals, Delhi 110092).
4. Benzyl benzoate application (Rays Labs. Pvt. Ltd., Calcutta 700007).

Lotions

Lotions are usually suspensions or dispersions intended for external application to the skin. They are applied directly to the skin without rubbing with the help of some absorbent material such as cotton wool or the cotton wool or gauze soaked in the lotion is applied to the affected part. Lotions may be employed for local cooling, soothing or protective purposes. Dermatologists frequently prescribe lotions for anaesthetic or antiseptic actions. The inclusion of alcohol in a lotion hastens its drying and produces cooling effect whereas the addition of glycerin in a lotion keeps the skin moist for sufficiently long time and does not allow the preparation to dry.

Bacterias and molds grow in certain lotions if no preservative is added to the preparation. Even if a preservative is added care must be taken to avoid contamination during preparation of the lotion.

Lotions should be dispensed in coloured fluted bottles in order to distinguish from preparations meant for internal use. The container should be labelled "For external use only.". On long standing the lotions have a tendency to separate out. Therefore, the container must be labelled "Shake before use.".

Examples are calamine lotion, oily calamine lotion, salicylic acid lotion and zinc sulphate lotion.

Lotions Containing Insoluble Substances

When a lotion contains insoluble substances of indiffusible nature, it will have to be dispensed in lotions like that of mixtures, i.e., by incorporating a suspending agent. For this purpose gummy suspending agents like tragacanth is not suitable because of their sticky nature. Therefore, bentonite and aluminium hydroxide gel are sometimes used as suspending agents.

Calamine lotion is the best example of lotions containing insoluble substances. This lotion contains calamine, zinc oxide, bentonite, sodium citrate, liquefied phenol, glycerin and purified water.

Here calamine is an insoluble substance of indiffusible nature. It acts as astringent, soothing and protective agent. Zinc oxide is an adjuvant, it acts as mild astringent with local soothing, protective and antiseptic properties. Bentonite acts as a suspending agent which swells up in water and imparts viscosity to the solution. Sodium citrate is incorporated to prevent the lotion from being too viscous. Liquefied phenol is used as an antiseptic and glycerin as a humectant.

Method of Preparation

Triturate calamine, zinc oxide and bentonite with a portion of sodium citrate solution in a mortar till a smooth cream is formed. Add remaining amount of sodium citrate solution and mix well. Incorporate glycerin and liquefied phenol, mix thoroughly. Add more of vehicle to produce the required volume. Stir thoroughly so as to get a homogeneous product.

Rx

Calamine	15.0 gm
Zinc oxide	5.0 gm
Bentonite	3.0 gm
Sodium citrate	0.5 gm
Liquefied phenol	0.5 ml
Glycerin	5.0 ml
Purified water up to	100.0 ml

Make : Lotion. Send 50 ml.

Direction : To be applied to the affected part of the skin without friction.

Procedure

Mix the weighed amount of calamine, zinc oxide and bentonite in a mortar. Triturate it with a solution of sodium citrate in about 70 ml of purified water. Add the required quantity of liquefied phenol and glycerin. Mix well. To this add more of vehicle to produce the required volume. Mix thoroughly so as to get a uniform preparation. Transfer to a bottle, cork, label and dispense. Apply the secondary label "Shake the bottle before use." and "For external use only.".

Uses

This lotion is used as an astringent and protectant from sunburn. It acts as a soothening agent and gives relief from itching and pain during skin irritation. It is also used in ringworm infection and eczema.

1. Calamine is basic zinc carbonate mixed with suitable amount of ferric oxide to impart pink colour. It is often prescribed by dermatologists to give flesh like colour to lotions or creams.
2. Zinc oxide has mild astringent, protective and antiseptic action. It is widely used in dusting powders, lotion, and ointments meant for the treatment of skin diseases and infections such as eczema, ringworm, psoriasis (chronic skin disease in which red scaly patches develop) and pruritus (itching).

3. Bentonite is a native colloidal hydrated aluminium silicate. It is insoluble in water but swells up nearly seven times its bulk and forms a magma with desirable viscosity. Hence it is used as suspending agent for the dispersion of insoluble substances like calamine, etc.
4. Sodium citrate is added to prevent the lotion from being too viscous. It acts as a buffer and maintains the pH appropriate for skin preparations.
5. Liquefied phenol acts as antipruritic because of its antiseptic properties and also because of its local anaesthetic action.
6. Glycerin acts as a hygroscopic thus keeps the skin moist and have soothening effect on the skin.

Marketed Lotions

1. Caladryl lotion [Parke-Davis (India) Ltd., Bombay - 400025].

Contains :

Calamine	8%	w/v
Camphor	0.1%	w/v
Diphenhydramine HCl	1%	w/v
Special denatured spirit	2.37%	v/v

2. Calderm skin lotion (Dermocare Labs, Ahmedabad - 380001).

Contains :

Calamine	15% w/w
Zinc oxide	5% w/w
Glycerin	5% w/w

3. Calamine lotion (Alpine Industries, New Delhi - 110028).

Each contains :

Calamine	160 gm
Zinc oxide	50 gm
Bentonite	30 gm
Sod. citrate	5 gm
Liquefied phenol	5 ml
Glycerin	50 ml
Rose water	1000 ml

4. Calamine lotion [Jilichem Labs (India) Ltd., Ahmedabad - 382445].
5. Calamine lotion (Agrawal Pharmaceuticals, Delhi - 110092).
6. Senee hair lotion (Dermocare Labs, Ahmedabad - 380001).

Revision Questions

I. Very short answer type questions

Define the following :

(A)

(i) Monophasic liquid dosage forms.
(ii) Solutions
(iii) Mixtures
(iv) Draught
(v) Solubility
(vi) Supersaturated solutions
(vii) Diffusible solids
(viii) Indiffusible solids
(ix) Liniments
(x) Lotions

(B) Fill in the blanks :

(a) Liquids for external use are dispensed in coloured ...... bottles.
(b) Simple syrup contains ...... percent sucrose.
(c) Bottles containing liniments and Lotions must be ...... before use.
(d) Liniments must not be applied on the ...... skin.
(e) Compound tragacanth powder is used as suspending agent in the ratio of ...... of total mixture to be prepared.

II. Short answer type questions

1. What are monophasic liquid dosage forms? Explain the advantages and disadvantages of liquid dosage forms.
2. Explain the following :
   (i) Why glycerin is used as a base is throat paints?
   (ii) Why liniments should not be rubbed on broken skin?
   (iii) Why gargles are dispensed in concentrated form?
   (iv) Why linctuses should be sipped and not swallowed?
   (v) Why oily vehicle is not used in the preparation of nasal drops?
3. Write short notes on the followings :
   (i) Solubilization
   (ii) Co-solvency
   (iii) Complexation
   (iv) Hydrotrophy
   (v) Liniments
   (vi) Lotions
   (vii) Syrups
   (viii) Elixirs
   (ix) Gargles
   (x) Mouthwashes
   (xi) Douches
   (xii) Enemas
   (xiii) Throat paints

(xiv) Ear drops

(xv) Sprays

4. Differentiate the following :
   (a) Syrups and elixirs
   (b) Drops and draughts
   (c) Liniments and Lotions
   (d) Gargles and mouth washes
   (e) Throat paints and sprays
   (f) Enemas and douches
   (g) Nasal drops and inhalations
   (h) Eye drops and eye lotions.

III. Long answer type questions :

1. What are solutions? Explain the advantages and disadvantages of solutions over other dosage form of drugs. Describe how solutions differ from mixtures.
2. What do you understand by the term solubility? Discuss various techniques of enhancing solubility of drugs in vehicles.
3. Define solubility discuss in detail the methods of increasing the solubility with examples.
4. Discuss briefly the problems, which are encountered during the formulation of monophonic liquid dosage form of drugs.
5. What are mixtures? Describe the general method of dispensing of :
   (a) Mixtures containing diffusible solids.
   (b) Mixtures containing indiffusible solids.
   (c) Mixtures containing precipitate forming liquids.
6. Classify monophasic liquids for internal administration. What type of colours, flavours and sweeteners are used for such formulations.
7. Classify monophasic liquids for external use. Discuss liniments in detail.
8. What are lotions? How would you dispense lotions containing insoluble substances?
9. Give at least three examples of marketed preparations of the following pharmaceuticals :

(a) Mixtures/liquid preparations	(b) Solutions
(c) Syrups	(d) Drops
(e) Expectorants	(f) Drops
(g) Mouth washes and gargles	(h) Throat paints
(i) Ear drops	(j) Nasal drops
(k) Liniments	(l) Lotions

Answers

(a) Flutted; (b) 66.7 W/W; (c) Shaken; (d) Broken; (c) 2%

6

Additives in Dosage Forms

Additives are the substances other than the active medicament(s) in the formulation which do not have any pharmacological action. They are used to give a particular shape to the formulation, to increase the stability and/or to increase the palatability and elegance of the preparation. Additives may be exemplified by surfactants, hydrocolloids, diluents, vehicles, bases, stabilizers, preservatives, colouring agents, flavouring agents and sweetening agents, etc. Some of the formulations may contain all the additives but others may contain one or more than one additive. They should be used very carefully so that they may not interfere with the therapeutic activity of the active medicament and does not affect the stability of the preparation.

Surfactants

Surfactants or surface active agents are one of the most important classes of additives which are used in pharmaceutical formulations. Due to one reason or the other they are used in almost all liquid, semisolid or solid formulations. They may be used as emulsifying agents, detergents, solubilising agents, wetting agents, foaming agents, antifoaming agents, flocculating agents and deflocculating agents.

Surfactants may be defined as the substances which when added to a liquid, lower the interfacial tension between two phases, thus make them miscible with each other. This phenomenon is commonly used to make two immiscible liquids miscible with each other and to dissolve the drugs which are normally insoluble in aqueous vehicles.

The molecules of a surfactant consist of two parts, i.e., a polar part and non-polar part. When such molecules are placed in two phases of different polarities the polar part moves towards high polarity phase while non-polar part moves towards the low polarity phase and preferentially they are absorbed at the interphase. As the concentration is increased, a level is reached where the interphase becomes saturated with surface active agents and no more space is available at the surface to be occupied, therefore the surfactant molecules move towards the bulk of the solution. At this concentration an unusual phenomenon occurs. The molecules tend to form colloidal aggregates known as micelles consisting of 50 to 150 molecules of surface active agents. The concentration of surfactant at which the micelles are formed is known as critical micelle concentration or C.M.C. The solubilization begins at C.M.C. and generally increases with increase in the concentration of micelles.

Classification of Surfactants

Surfactants may be classified in a number of ways depending on the use and physical or chemical properties but the most widely accepted system of classification is based on their ionic behaviour in solutions which is explained as follows :

(a) **Anionics/anion active surfactants :** They ionise in aqueous solutions into a large anion which is responsible for their emulsifying ability. Examples are soaps of monovalent and divalent metals, sulphated compounds like sodium lauryl sulphate, sodium cetyl sulphate, sulfonated compounds like dioctyl sodium sulfosuccinate, etc.

(b) **Cationics/cation active surfactants :** They ionise in aqueous solutions into a large cation, responsible for their emulsifying ability. Examples are benzylkonium chloride, cetyl trimethyl ammonium bromide, etc.

(c) **Non-ionic surfactants :** They do not ionise in aqueous solutions. Examples are glyceryl monostearate, spans and tweens. This is the most widely used class of surfactants in pharmaceutical industries because they offer a wide range of physical properties and are stable over a wide range of pH.

Hydrocolloids

Hydrocolloids are the high molecular weight solid substances which when added to water produce highly viscous solutions, suspensions or gels. They are also known as gums and consist of polysaccharides, and proteins. Most of the water soluble hydrocolloids are more soluble in hot water than in cold water and tend to precipitate or form gel on cooling, e.g., agar and gelatin. Certain water-soluble polymers like methyl cellulose, hydroxy propyl cellulose are more soluble in cold water than in hot water. Their solutions tend to gel on heating.

Classification

Hydrocolloids may be classified as follows :

(a) Natural
(b) Semi-synthetic
(c) Synthetic.

(a) Natural

Naturally occuring hydrocolloids may be obtained from plants, animals and minerals. Hydrocolloids obtained from plants are most widely used and are known as gums which consist of polysaccharides. They are very commonly used in textile, paper, food, cosmetic, pharmaceutical and other industries. The hydrocolloids obtained from plants include acacia, tragacanth, agar, etc. Gelatin and casein are the examples of hydrocolloids obtained from animals. The mineral hydrocolloids include colloidal silica, colloidal alumina, bentonite and veegum.

(b) Semi-Synthetic Hydrocolloids

They are the substances which are produced by chemical modification of cellulose obtained from wood, pulp or cotton to produce soluble polymers. The modified derivatives so produced have many advantages over the parent molecules. Some of the hydrocolloids produced in this way are methylcellulose, sodium carboxymethyl cellulose, hydroxyethyl cellulose and hydroxypropyl cellulose.

(c) Synthetic Hydrocolloids

A number of hydrocolloids have been synthesised but only a few are used in pharmaceutical formulations, e.g., carbopols and polyox.

Vehicles

A vehicle may be described as a medium in which the ingredients of a formulation are dissolved, suspended or dispersed for their easy administration and rapid pharmacological action. The vehicle is a loose word which may be used for liquids, semisolids or solids. When a liquid is used to dissolve or suspend the medicament, the liquid is known as vehicle whereas when semisolid or solid is used to disperse the medicament, it is known as base. Vehicles may also by used to increase the bulk of the preparation. The commonly used vehicles in pharmaceutical formulations are described below :

1. Water

Water is the most suitable choice of vehicle because it can dissolve a large number of drugs and they can be easily administered to the body as it does not interfere with the metabolic reactions.

When water is required as vehicle for oral preparations, potable water or purified water should be used. Sometimes, potable water contains dissolved impurities and micro-organisms therefore it should be made free from impurities and must be freshly boiled and cooled to destroy the micro-organisms.

2. Aromatic Waters

Sometimes aromatic waters are used as vehicles mainly due to their flavouring properties. Some of them possess mild therapeutic and/or preservative properties. The commonly used aromatic waters are chloroform water, camphor water, cinnamon water, peppermint water, anise water and dill water.

3. Infusions

Some of the infusions which have definite therapeutic properties are prescribed as vehicles. They include compound gentian infusion, orange peel infusion, senega infusion and infusion of clove.

4. Water for Injection

Whenever water is to be used as vehicle in injectable preparations, distilled water free from pyrogens must be used. Water is used as the vehicle for most of injectable preparations because aqueous preparations are tolerated well by the body and are the safest and easiest to administer.

5. Alcohol

Alcohol is considered a very good solvent which comes next in importance to water. It has an advantage over water that preparations made with it remain stable for quite a long time because of its antimicrobial properties, while many aqueous solutions of organic substances soon hydrolyse and become unfit for use. Water and alcohol are quite miscible with each other and can be mixed in any proportions. Such mixtures of water and alcohol are referred to as hydroalcoholic solvents which are extensively used in pharmaceutical formulations.

6. Glycerin

Glycerin is an excellent solvent but it is not as commonly used as that of water or alcohol. It is a polyhydric alcohol which is quite viscous and hygroscopic in nature. Because of its viscous nature glycerin is an essential ingredient of throat paints so that the medicament should remain in contact with mucous membrane of the throat for a longer time. Due to humectant properties, glycerin is used in creams, jellies, paints, lotions and other preparations meant for external application to the skin.

7. Propylene Glycol

Propylene glycol is widely used as a substitute for glycerin. It is miscible with water, acetone and chloroform in all proportions. It can dissolve many volatile oils but fixed oils are insoluble in it.

8. Oils

Oils obtained from vegetable and animal kingdom are frequently used as solvents for pharmaceutical preparations. Vegetable oils like castor oil, cottonseed oil and corn oil are commonly used but they are decreasing in favour because they easily get rancid and develop bacterial growth on storage. They differ greatly in their qualities because they are obtained from natural origin. Due to these reasons vegetable oils are being replaced with mineral oils like liquid paraffin because it is quite stable and free from odour and taste. But liquid paraffin or solid paraffin cannot be used in parenteral preparations because they would not be metabolised by the body tissues and may develop tissue reactions and even tumours. Therefore oils are generally used in preparations meant for external use.

Some newer non-aqueous vehicles are recently developed which are used in the formulation of parenteral preparations and they are found more satisfactory than vegetable and mineral oils. Among these are polyethylene glycols, isopropyl myristate, etc.

Bases

The term base is used for semisolid and solid substances in which the drug is incorporated either to increase the bulk or to give a particular shape to the dosage form. Generally these types of bases are used for the preparation of ointments and suppositories where they are known as ointment bases and suppository bases respectively. These types of bases do not merely carry the medicaments but exert great influence over their pharmacological actions. The rate of absorption of a drug through the skin mainly depends on the nature of ointment base used in the formulation of ointments. An ideal ointment base should be non-irritant, easily applicable, easily removable, compatible with medicaments and skin secretions and should release the incorporated medicament readily. The commonly used ointment bases are soft paraffin, hard paraffin, liquid paraffin, wool fat, wool alcohol, bees wax, etc.

Since the suppositories are special shaped solid dosage form of medicament they must retain its shape, solidity and firmness during storage and administration but must melt or dissolve in the cavity fluids when inserted into the body cavity. Therefore the materials used as suppository bases must impart these properties and also fulfil other formulation requirements. There are a large number of bases used but theobroma oil, glycerogelatin and polyethylene glycols fulfils the above mentioned requirements. Coconut oil, stearin, hydrogenated peanut oil and mixture of oleic acid and stearic acid in combination with some waxes have also been recommended as suppository bases.

Diluents

Diluents are the inert substances which are specially added to increase the bulk of a drug or to decrease its concentration. The liquids which are used as vehicles may be specifically used as diluents but for oral preparations water is the most suitable diluent.

Solid diluents are included in the formulation of powders, granules, capsules and tablets, etc., where they are used to increase the bulk of other materials for easy conversion into proper dosage form. In potent drugs, diluents are incorporated to increase the bulk so that they can be weighed easily and divided conveniently into required number of doses.

The diluent used must be inert, compatible with other ingredients of the formulation, physically and chemically stable and should not affect the bioavailability of the drug. There are a large number of substances available which can be used as diluents but lactose is the most suitable and widely used diluent for oral preparations. Other diluents which are used include sucrose, sorbitol, mannitol, wheat starch, corn starch, rice starch, potato starch, and microcrystalline cellulose. Some salts like dibasic calcium phosphate, calcium sulphate and sodium chloride, etc., can also be used as diluents.

The diluents incorporated in the formulations meant of external use include talc, kaolin, starch, etc. Talc is the most widely used diluent in dusting powders because apart from diluent action, it imparts necessary spreading characteristics to the dusting powders. Whenever talc is used as diluent, sterilized talc free from cl. tetani must be used.

Stabilizers

Stability of pharmaceutical product may be defined as the capability of a particular formulation in a specific container to remain within the physical, chemical, microbiogical, therapeutic and toxicological specifications. The substances which are used to control these stabilities are known as stabilizers. The most important stabilizers are the antioxidants and preservatives.

(a) Antioxidants

An antioxidant is a substance which is added to pharmaceutical formulation to prevent the oxidative degradation of the drug. The antioxidants have great affinity for oxygen and when they are added to formulation they compete for it affording protection to other oxygen sensitive drugs.

An ideal antioxidant should be stable and effective against a wide range of pH, colourless, nontoxic, nonirritant, thermostable and compatible with formulation ingredients and packaging material. Some of the commonly used antioxidants are sodium bisulfite, sodium metabisulfite, sodium thiosulphate, ascorbic acid, ascorbyl palmitate hydroquinone, propyl gallate, butylated hydroxy toluene, butylated hydroxyanisole and tocopherols.

(b) Preservatives

A preservative is a substance which is added to pharmaceutical formulations to prevent or inhibit the growth of microorganisms in the preparations. They are added to all formulations which are to be stored for long periods of time and the ingredients of which support microbial growth. The emulsions and suspensions containing water and carbohydrates as emulsifying and suspending agents respectively, must be suitably preserved because water and carbohydrates provide very good medium for the multiplication of bacterias and molds. Further, the parenteral preparations packed in multidose containers must contain a preservative to check the growth of microorganisms which may have accidentally entered the container during the withdrawal of a dose.

A preservative is unnecessary in multidose containers prepared by heating with bactericide because they already contain a lethal substance, nor they are necessary in preparations which contain medicaments having bactericidal properties.

Choice of Preservative

The preservative selected should have the following properties :

1. It should be effective against a wide range of microorganisms.
2. It should be compatible with other ingredients of the formulation.
3. It should be soluble in aqueous phase when used in emulsions.
4. It should be nontoxic.
5. It should be free from odour and taste.
6. It should preserve the preparations and remain stable for the shelf life of the product.

No single preservative possesses all the qualities therefore it becomes necessary to use a combination of preservatives to prevent the growth of microorganisms. The most commonly used preservatives are as follows :

1. Benzoic acid and sodium benzoate 0.1 to 0.2%.
2. Salicylic acid 0.1%.
3. Phenol 0.2 to 0.5%.
4. Chlorocresol 0.05 to 0.1%.
5. Alcohol 15 to 20%.
6. Chlorbutanol 0.5%.
7. Phenylmercuric nitrate 0.002 to 0.005%.
8. Sorbic acid and its salts 0.05 to 0.2%.
9. Benzalkonium chloride 0.004 to 0.02%.
10. Methyl paraben and propyl paraben 0.1% to 0.2%.

Colouring Agents

Colouring agents may be defined as the substances used to impart colour to foods, drugs and cosmetics to increase their organoleptic properties. In pharmaceutical preparations they may be used to increase their acceptability by the patients, to give warning, or to produce standard preparations.

Colours may be obtained from minerals, plants and animals or they can be prepared by synthesis. Colours obtained from minerals are also known as pigments. At one time they were used in cosmetics and lotions meant for external application to the skin but now a days their use is restricted and are replaced by synthetic colours. The examples of mineral colours are ferric oxide (yellow and red), carbon black, titanium dioxide and ultramarine.

Different colours obtained from plants include chlorophyll, indigo, alizarin, carotenoids and flavones. Cochineal was the only animal colour used in pharmaceutical preparations. But now a days the colours obtained from plants and animals are rarely used, they are replaced by synthetic colours.

The synthetic colours are prepared from coal tar dyes which include nitro-dyes, nitroso-dyes, azo-dyes, thiazines, rosanilines, etc. They are mainly used in textile industries. Only the permitted colours are used in food and pharmaceutical preparations. Caramel or burnt sugar, an artificial colour is used to produce brown colour in cough syrups, elixirs and other oral liquid preparations.

Amount of Colouring Agent Required

There is no hard and fast rule regarding the quantity of colouring agent used in the preparations. It depends upon the depth of colour required, the thickness of solution to be viewed and the presence of suspended powders in the preparation. An approximate quantity of colouring agent used for liquid preparations is 0.0001% to 0.001% and for powders is 0.1%.

Flavouring Agents

Flavouring agents are the substances which are used to impart pleasant smell to the preparation and to mask specific type of taste of the preparation, thus make them more palatable. Most of the flavours used in pharmaceutical preparations are obtained from natural sources but now a days they are being replaced by synthetic flavours.

There are a large number of flavouring agents which are used to impart acceptable smell to pharmaceutical preparations. Generally the preparations which are taken orally are flavoured with fruity and spicy flavours and the preparations which are applied externally are flavoured with flowery flavouring agents. The flavouring agents obtained from natural sources include pine-apple, banana, cardamom, ginger, cinnamom, peppermint and volatile oils obtained from anise, caraway, clove, dill, lemon, orange, rose, jasmine, lavender, etc. Malt extract, glycyrrihiza extract, coffee, vanilla, chocolate and tolu balsam are also used as flavouring agents. Menthol, mannitol, chloroform spirit and chloroform water are widely used as flavouring agents in liquid formulations.

Synthetic chemicals like certain alcohols, aldehydes, esters, fatty acids, ketones and lactones are used as flavouring agents. They are often preferred to natural flavouring agents because :

(i) they are constant in composition;
(ii) they are readily available;
(iii) they are comparatively cheap;
(iv) they are more stable;
(v) their incompatibilities are more predictable.

Selection of Flavours

The problem of selection of a flavour for a particular preparation is quite complicated because flavour and taste depends on individual preferences. Moreover it depends on the qualities of the preparation which is to be flavoured. For salty preparations, cinnamon flavours are considered the best flavouring agents followed by orange syrup, cocoa syrup, wild cherry syrup and raspberry syrup. For bitter taste cocoa syrup, raspberry syrup, cherry syrup and cinnamon syrup are used. The acrid taste and sour taste can be masked by raspberry and other fruit syrups.

Oily taste of fixed oil like that of castor oil can be effectively masked with aromatic rhubarb syrup and that of cod-liver oil can be masked by oil of winter green, peppermint oil, malt extract or glycyrrihiza extract.

A blend of flavouring agents is generally used to effectively mask the odour and taste sensations. As regards the quantities of flavouring agents used in formulations, it mainly depends on the formulator. Usually 0.1 to 0.5% of volatile oil is sufficient as flavouring agent for an emulsion.

Sweetening Agents

Sweetening agents are the substances which are used in the formulations to mask the objectionable taste of the drug and make the preparation sweet in taste. Sucrose is the most widely used sweetening agent. It is obtained from sugar cane. It is quite soluble in water. It is physically and chemically stable at pH from 4.0 to 8.0. Simple syrup and liquid glucose are frequently used in liquid preparations. Sugar is also used in lozenges and in the coating of pills and tablets. The other sweetening agents include lactose, mannitol, honey, glycerin and sorbitol.

Artificial or synthetic sweetening agents like saccharin, sodium saccharin and sodium cyclamate are frequently used in the preparation of sugar free formulations. These compounds are soluble in water, alcohol and glycols. They are physically and chemically stable over a pH range of 3.0 to 8.0. A desired sweetness can be produced at much lower concentration than sucrose. Saccharin in dilute solutions is 300 times as sweet as sucrose. Saccharin sodium is used in tooth pastes and other preparations meant for oral hygiene because it is less likely to cause dental carries than carbohydrates. It is also used as a sweetening agent for many foods for diabetic persons and those who are on slimming diets.

Revision Questions

I. Very short answer type questions

Define the following :

(a) Additives

(b) Surfactants
(c) Hydrocolloids
(d) Vehicles
(e) Bases
(f) Diluents
(g) Stabilizers
(h) Antioxidants
(i) Preservatives
(j) Colouring agents
(k) Flavouring agents
(l) Sweetening agents

II. Short answer type questions

Write short notes on the following

1. Surfactants
2. Hydrocolloids
3. Vehicles
4. Bases
5. Diluents
6. Stabilizers
7. Antioxidants
8. Preservatives
9. Colouring agents
10. Flavouring agents
11. Sweetening agents

III. Long answer type questions

1. What do you understand by the term 'additives'? Enumerate various additives used in the formulation of drugs. Illustrate your answer by giving suitable examples.
2. Describe the terms 'surfactants' and 'hydrochlorides'. Classify and explain different types of surfactants and hydrochlorides used in pharmaceutical formulations.
3. Differentiate between the following :
   (a) Surfactants and hydrochlorides.
   (b) Vehicles and bases.
   (c) Preservatives and antioxidants.
   (d) Flavouring agents and sweetening agents.

4. What are stabilizers? Give their uses in pharmaceutical industry.
5. Define the terms 'colouring agents' Flavouring agents and sweetening agents. Describe the necessity of adding such agents in pharmaceutical formulations.

7

Suspensions

Suspensions are the biphasic liquid dosage form of medicament in which the finely divided solid particles ranging from 0.5 to 5.0 micron are suspended or dispersed in a liquid or semi-solid vehicle. The solid particles constitutes the discontinuous phase whereas the liquid vehicle constitutes the continuous phase. Suspensions are mainly used for oral administration, external application or parenteral use. Oral suspensions can be made more palatable by using derivative of the drug as in the case of chloramphenicol palmitate. Suspensions are also chemically more stable than solutions. That is why now a days many suspensions are marketed as dry powders and the patient or pharmacist is asked to incorporate a specified amount of the vehicle to constitute the suspension before its use. Suspension is an ideal dosage form for patients who cannot swallow tablets or capsules. Suspensions meant for external application should have very small particle size to avoid gritty feeling to the skin. Similarly suspensions meant for introduction into the ophthalmic cavity should be free from gritty particles to avoid irritation, pain and discomfort. In some cases, sterile suspensions are injected hypodermically to produce sustained action of the drug which will not be produced by a true solution of the same drug.

Qualities of Good Suspension

A well formulated suspension should have the following properties :

1. The dispersed particles should not settle readily and the settled particles should redisperse immediately on shaking.
2. The particles should not form a cake on settling.
3. The viscosity should be such that the preparation can be easily poured.
4. It should be chemically stable.
5. Suspensions for internal use must be palatable and suspensions for external use must be free from gritty particles and possess other characteristics required for external preparations.

Flocculated and Non-Flocculated Suspensions

In flocculated suspensions the individual particles are in contact with each other to form loose aggregates and create a network like structure. Although the rate of sedimentation is high but the sediment is loosely packed which can redisperse easily on shaking so as to reform the original suspension. However the flocculated suspensions meant for oral, parenteral, ophthalmic or external use may not be elegant because they are difficult to remove from bottles or vials and on transferring from the bottle the floccules remain sticking to the sides of the bottle. These properties can be improved by adding protective colloids.

In non-flocculated or de-flocculated suspensions all individual particles exist as separate entities. The rate of sedimentation is slow and a sediment is formed slowly but the sediment is closely packed due to weight of upper layers of sedimenting materials. A hard cake is formed which is difficult to redisperse to get original suspension. The non-flocculated suspensions have pleasing appearance as compared to flocculated suspensions because the substances remain suspended for a sufficiently long time.

Relative Properties of Flocculated and Non-Flocculated Suspensions

	Flocculated	*Non-Flocculated*
1.	Particles form loose aggregates and form a network like structure.	Particles exist as separate entities.
2.	Rate of sedimentation is high.	Rate of sedimentation is slow.
3.	Sediment is rapidly formed.	Sediment is slowly formed.
4.	Sediment is loosely packed and does not form a hard cake.	Sediment is very closely packed and a hard cake is formed.
5.	Sediment is easy to redisperse.	Sediment is difficult to redisperse.
6.	Suspension is not pleasing in appearance.	Suspension is pleasing in appearance.
7.	The floccules stick to the sides of the bottle.	They do not stick to the sides of the bottle.

Formulation of Suspensions

Before selecting the additives to be used in the formulation of suspensions it is very important to decide whether the particles in suspension are to be flocculated or to remain non-flocculated. Following are the additives which are generally used in the formulation of suspensions :

1. Flocculating agents
2. Suspending agents/thickening agents
3. Wetting agents

4. Dispersing agents
5. Preservative
6. Organoleptic additives.

1. Flocculating Agents

When formulating suspensions it must be ensured that the particles are well dispersed in the vehicle. The dispersion can be improved by adding a surfactant which will act by reducing the interfacial tension. For example, if surfactants with negative charges are adsorbed on the particles, prevents or minimises flocculation in the presence of positive ions because of natural repulsion of like charges. Sodium lauryl sulphate and sodium dioctyl sulphosuccinate are examples of this type of surfactants. Non-ionic surfactants also usually assume a negative charge in solution thereby act as effective flocculating agents. Generally non-ionic surfactants are used for dispersing the insoluble particles. Tweens, spans and carbowaxes are frequently used in this manner.

Protective colloids can also be used as flocculating agents. They differ from surfactants in that they do not reduce the interfacial tension. Their solutions differ in viscosity and are used in higher concentration than surfactants.

2. Suspending Agents/Thickening Agents

Suspending agents are the substances which are added to a suspension to increase the viscosity of the continuous phase so that the particles remain suspended for a sufficiently long time and it becomes easy to measure an accurate dose.

While selecting a suspending agent it is not only important that it should increase the viscosity of the system but the pourability, spreadability, etc., of the final product must also be taken into consideration. Some of the thickening agents used in formulations include acacia, tragacanth and sodium alginate. As these are natural products therefore vary in qualities and properties hence not very commonly used. The semi-synthetic thickening agents widely used include methyl cellulose, carboxy methyl cellulose, hydroxypropyl methyl cellulose, synthetic polymers and gelatin. Sodium carboxy methyl cellulose in concentration of about 3.5% is used in injectable suspensions. Clays such as hydrated aluminium silicate or magnesium silicate are also used as suspending agents. Non-ionic substances such as sorbitol, glycerin, sugar or polyethylene glycols may be included to adjust the viscosity of the medium.

3. Wetting Agents

Wetting agents are the substances which reduce the interfacial tension between the solid particles and liquid medium thus producing a suspension of desired quality. This may be achieved by adding a suitable wetting agent which is adsorbed at the solid/liquid interface in such a way that the affinity of the particles for the surrounding medium is increased and the interparticular forces are decreased. Examples of wetting agents are alcohol in tragacanth mucilage, glycerin and glycols in sodium alginate or bentonite dispersions and polysorbates in oral and parenteral suspensions.

Only a minimum amount of wetting agent should be used; excessive amounts may lead to foaming or impart an undesirable taste or odour to the suspension.

4. Dispersing Agents

The first step in the formulation of any suspension is to ensure that the particles are dispersed in and wetted by the dispersion medium. In some substances where the surface energy is not sufficient the particles may come together and form larger particles. To overcome this difficulty the substances which are used are known as dispersing agents. They carry good charge and are easily adsorbed on to the disperse phase particles. These substances increase the zeta potential and do not allow the particles to come together to form large particles.

5. Preservative

The presence of suspending agents and medicaments which are liable for bacterial growth makes it necessary to incorporate a preservative in suspensions. Preservatives selected should be effective against a wide range of micro-organisms and should be chemically and physically stable. It should be non-toxic and compatible with other added substances. The commonly used preservatives are benzoic acid, sodium benzoate, methyl paraben and propyl-paraben.

6. Organoleptic Additives

Colours, sweetening agents and flavouring agents are used in oral suspensions. Similarly colours and perfumes are incorporated in suspensions meant for external application but these must be compatible with other ingredients.

Preparation of Suspensions

These preparations are generally of two types :

1. Those in which the insoluble substances are added to the vehicle or the vehicle is added to the insoluble substances.
2. Those in which the insoluble material is formed in the liquid due to the interaction of two or more ingredients.

Some of the preparations can be made by both of these methods, others by only one method but most of the preparations containing insoluble materials are prepared by the first method, i.e., by adding the insoluble material to the vehicle.

(a) Suspensions Containing Diffusible Solids

Diffusible solids are those substances which do not dissolve in water, but on shaking they can be mixed with it and remain evenly distributed throughout the liquid for sufficiently long time allowing uniform distribution of the drug in each dose. However, on standing, the insoluble solids settle at the bottom of the bottle which require re-shaking of the bottle each time whenever a dose is to be measured. Hence the bottle containing the diffusible mixture must be labelled "Shake the bottle before use.". Diffusible solids include aromatic chalk powder, bismuth carbonate, light kaolin, magnesium oxide, light magnesium carbonate, heavy magnesium carbonate, magnesium trisilicate, phenolphthalein, rhubarb powder.

Method of Dispensing

Finely powder the diffusible and other substances (if they are already not in fine powder) in a mortar. Mix them thoroughly. Add a small amount of vehicle out of ¾th measured out vehicle and triturate to make a smooth cream. (Due to the presence of air in the interstices of many powders, they float at the surface of water and do not mix with the vehicle. To prevent this tendency, a smooth cream is prepared by adding a small amount of vehicle at first and then diluted.) Add the remainder of vehicle. If foreign particles are visible pass the suspension through a piece of muslin but if one or two foreign particles are visible, remove them with a glass rod. Add liquid ingredients and make up the required volume by adding more of vehicle. Transfer the suspension to a bottle, cork, polish, label and dispense. "Shake the bottle before use." label must be attached.

Rx

Light kaolin	2.0 gm
Light magnesium carbonate	0.5 gm
Sodium bicarbonate	0.5 gm
Peppermint water q.s.	15.0 ml

Make a mixture. Send six doses.

Direction : One dose to be taken three times a day.

Type : Mixture containing diffusible solids.

(b) Suspensions Containing Indiffusible Solids

Indiffusible solids are those substances which do not dissolve in water an do not remain evenly distributed in the vehicle for sufficiently long tim to ensure uniformity of the measured dose. This difficulty is overcome b increasing the viscosity of the vehicle for which purpose suspending agent are used. The two commonly used suspending agents are (a) compoun tragacanth powder which is used in the ratio of 2 gm per 100 ml of th suspension or 10 grain per ounce of the suspension to be prepare (b) tragacanth mucilage, it is used in the ratio of ¼th of the volume the suspension to be prepared. Tragacanth mucilage is used only when the vehicle is chloroform water or water because mucilage is prepared by using chloroform water and if added to preparations containing medicinally active vehicle may replace some of the medicinally active vehicle thereby decreasing their activity. In such cases compound tragacanth powder must be used as suspending agent. Indiffusible solids include : for oral suspensions — aspirin, aromatic chalk powder, phenobarbitone, succinyl sulphathiazole, sulphadimidine; and for externally used suspensions — calamine, sulphur precipitated, zinc oxide.

For its preparation, finely powder the indiffusible substance in a mortar, add any soluble or diffusible solids and compound tragacanth powder or tragacanth mucilage and mix thoroughly. If only indiffusible substance is to be incorporated, mix it with compound tragacanth powder in a mortar. Add sufficient amount of vehicle and triturate so as to form a smooth cream. Then add more of vehicle to form a pourable liquid. Remove the foreign particles and proceed further as described under suspensions containing diffusible solids.

Rx

Succinyl sulphathiazole, in powder	1.0 gm
Light kaolin	0.6 gm
Compound tragacanth powder	0.1 gm
Raspberry syrup	2.0 ml
Benzoic acid solution	0.2 ml
Amaranth solution	0.1 ml
Chloroform water to produce	10.0 ml

Fiat mistura. Mitte 90 ml.

Signa : Cochleare amplum ter in die sumenda.

Type : Mixture containing indiffusible solids.

(c) Suspensions Produced by Chemical Reactions

In this type of preparation of suspensions the highly diluted solutions of the reacting substances are mixed together so as to form very finely divided precipitates that can be easily distributed throughout the liquid by shaking. Precipitates so formed are generally diffusible in nature therefore there is no need of adding any suspending agent. Zinc sulphide lotion B.P.C. is prepared in this way.

Suspensions Containing Precipitate-forming Liquids

Precipitate forming liquids include : compound benzoin tincture, benzoin tincture, lobelia ethereal tincture, myrrh tincture, tolu tincture. These liquids are not only insoluble in water but they form indiffusible precipitates particularly when salts are present. They contain resinous matter and when mixed with water lead to precipitation of the resin and may stick to the sides of the bottle which will be difficult to rediffuse by shaking. To prevent this tendency a suspending agent like compound tragacanth powder 2 gm/100 ml or tragacanth mucilage ¼th of the total volume to be prepared, will have to be incorporated.

1. Method of preparation using compound traganth powder

This method is very convenient when diffusible or indiffusible solids are also included in the prescription and must be used when the vehicle is water or medicinally active.

Finely powder any insoluble solid if already not in powder form and mix it with compound tragacanth powder in a mortar (If no solid ingredient is to be used then place the compound tragacanth powder alone in the mortar.) Measure out half of the vehicle and incorporate a small amount out of it to the powders with thorough trituration until a smooth cream is formed. Then add the remainder amount of the vehicle.

Measure the precipitate forming liquid in a dry measure and add it in a slow stream in the centre of the cream with rapid stirring. Pouring the sticky liquid on the pestle or the sides of the mortar must be avoided.

Dissolve the soluble ingredient (if present) in sufficient amount of vehicle out of remaining half of the vehicle. Add it slowly with constant stirring to the cream to avoid local high concentrations that might neutralize the effect of suspending agent.

Examine the contents of the mortar critically. If foreign particles are visible pass the suspension through a piece of muslin but if one or two foreign particles are visible remove them with a glass rod. Add more of vehicle to produce the final volume. Transfer the suspension to a bottle, cork, polish, label and dispense. "Shake the bottle before use." label must be attached.

2. Method of preparation using tragacanth mucilage

This method is more rapid than the first method and may be used when insoluble solids are absent and the vehicle used is water or chloroform water.

Mix the tragacanth mucilage with an equal volume of vehicle. Measure the precipitate-forming liquid in a dry measure and pour in the centre of the mucilage with constant stirring.

Dissolve any soluble substances in ¼th of the vehicle and add to the above mixture. Examine the contents critically and remove any foreign particles. Transfer the suspension to a bottle, cork, polish, label and dispense. "Shake the bottle before use." label must be attached.

Rx

Potassium iodide	4 gm
Lobelia ethereal tincture	16 ml

Stramonium tincture	32 ml
Chloroform water q.s.	180 ml

Fiat mistura.

Signa : Cochleare magnum quarter in die sumenda.

Type : Mixture containing precipitate forming liquid.

Theory

Lobelia ethereal tincture is a precipitate forming liquid so a suspending agent will have to be added. The vehicle is chloroform water and there are no insoluble substances present. Therefore follow the method for precipitate forming liquids using tragacanth mucilage as suspending agent. Potassium iodide must be added after dilution and with continuous stirring.

Packaging and Storage

Oral suspensions should be packaged in wide mouth containers so that they can be easily removed from them and without any delay. All the containers in which suspensions are filled should have sufficient space above the liquid to permit adequate shaking. They must be labelled "Shake well." and it must be ensured to shake the bottle each time when taking the dose so as to evenly distribute the particles throughout the vehicle.

Physical stability of suspensions is greatly affected by extremes of temperatures. Suspensions should be stored in a cool place but should not be kept in refrigerator which may damage the product. Freezing should be avoided which may lead to aggregation of the suspended particles.

Marketed Suspensions

1. Acemiz suspension (Lupin Laboratories Ltd., Bombay - 400098).

   Each 5 ml contains :

   Astemizole 5 mg

2. Bactrim suspension (Roche Products Ltd., Bombay - 400034).

   Each 5 ml contains :

   Trimethoprim 40 mg

   Sulphamethoxazole 200 mg

3. Chloramphenicol palmitate suspension (Klar Sehen Pvt. Ltd., Calcutta - 700026).

   Each 5 ml contains :

   Chloramphenicol palmitate eq. to Chloramphenicol 125 mg

4. Dependal-M suspension (Eskayef Limited, Bangalore - 560049).

   Each 5 ml contains :

   Furazolidone 25 mg

   Metronidazole 75 mg

5. Campicillin (paediatric) suspension (Cadila Laboratories Ltd., Ahmedabad - 380050).

   Each ml contains :

Ampicillin anhydrous	100 mg

6. Penetrin suspension (Cyanamid India Ltd., Lederle Division, Bombay - 400025).

   Each 5 ml contains :

Trimethoprim	40 mg
Sulphadimidine	200 mg

7. Septran suspension (Burroughs Wellcome India Ltd., Bombay - 400023).

   Each 5 ml contains :

Trimethoprim	40 mg
Sulphamethonazole	200 mg

8. Wormin suspension (Cadila Laboratories Ltd., Ahmedabad - 380050).

   Each 5 ml contains :

Mebendazole	100 mg

Revision Questions

I. Very short answer type questions

1. Define the following :
   (a) Biphasic liquid dosage form.
   (b) Suspensions
   (c) Flocculated suspensions
   (d) Non-flocculated suspensions
   (e) Suspending agents
2. Fill in the blanks :
   (a) The particle size of the suspended drug particles in a suspension should be in the range of ..... to ..... micron.

(b) The fine particle size of solids in suspension give a ...... rate of ....

(c) The suspensions which are required to be instilled into the ophthalmic cavity should be free from ....

(d) Some sterile suspensions are injected hypodermically to produce ...... of the drug.

(e) In flocculated suspensions the particles form ...... and form a ...... like structure.

(f) In non-flocculated suspensions the particles exist as ....

(g) Wetting agents are the substances, which reduce the ...... between the solid particles and liquid medium.

II. Short answer type questions

(a) Describe the qualities of a good suspension.
(b) Differentiate between a flocculated and non-flocculated suspension.
(c) Differentiate between suspension and emulsion.
(d) Write short notes on the following :
  (i) Suspensions
  (ii) Flocculating agents
  (iii) Suspending/thickening agents
  (iv) Wetting agents
  (v) Suspension containing diffusible solids.
  (vi) Give at least three examples of marketed suspensions.

III. Long answer type questions

1. What are suspensions? Describe the qualities of a good suspension. Discuss various additives used in the formulation of suspensions.
2. Define the term suspension. Discuss different types of suspensions.
3. What do you understand by the terms diffusible solids and indiffusible solids? Discuss methods of preparation of suspensions containing diffusible solids and indiffusible solids.

Answers

I. 2.

(a) 0.5 to 5 micron
(b) Faster dissolution
(c) Gritty particles

(d) Sustained action.
(e) Loose aggregates, network
(f) Separate entities
(g) Interfacial tension

8

Emulsions

An emulsion is a liquid preparation containing two immiscible liquids, one of which is dispersed as minute globules into the other. The liquid that is broken up into globules is called the dispersed phase or internal phase and the liquid in which the globules are dispersed is known as continuous or external phase. The globules remain dispersed only for a short time and separation takes place quickly upon standing. Therefore a third substance known as emulsifying agent is added to the system which forms a film around the globules of the dispersed phase thereby the globules remain scattered indefinitely in the continuous phase and a uniform, stable product is formed.

An emulsion may also be defined as a biphasic liquid dosage form of medicament in which two immiscible liquids (generally one of which is water and the other is some lipid or oil) are made miscible by the addition of a third substance known as emulgent or emulsifying agent.

Emulsions are widely used in pharmacy and medicine. They are used internally as well as externally. Certain medicinal agents having an unpleasant taste and odour can be made more palatable for oral administration in the form of emulsions, which are otherwise difficult to take, e.g., cod-liver oil, castor oil, etc. The activity of certain drugs can be increased and action can be prolonged by emulsifying the drug in a suitable vehicle. Sterile stable intravenous emulsions containing fats, carbohydrates and vitamins all in one preparation can be administered to the patients who are unable to take these vital substances by oral route. Dermatological preparations like creams and lotions are extensively formulated as emulsions. Most recently the foam aerosols have been developed in the form of emulsions.

Types of Emulsions

There are two types of emulsions :

(a) Oil in water type (O/W)
(b) Water in oil type (W/O).

In oil in water type emulsions the oil is in the dispersed phase whereas water is in the continuous phase. These types of emulsions are prepared by using emulsifying agents like gum acacia, tragacanth, methyl cellulose, saponins, synthetic substances and soaps formed from monovalent bases like Na^+, K^+ and NH_4^+. Oil in water type emulsions are preferred for internal use because the unpleasant taste and odour is masked by emulsification and oil being in a finely dispersed state is more quickly assimilated in the body.

In water in oil type emulsions, the water is in the dispersed phase whereas oil is in the continuous phase. These types of emulsions are mainly used externally as lotions or creams. Some oil in water type emulsions can also be used externally. The type of emulsifying agent used will determine the kind of emulsion formed. Antiseptics and other medicaments are more effective when used in the form of oil in water type emulsions. When an emollient action is required then water in oil emulsions are used externally. Emulsifying agents like wool fat, resins, bees wax, synthetic compounds and soaps formed from divalent bases like Ca^{++}, Mg^{++} and Zn^{++} are used for the preparation of water in oil emulsions.

Microemulsions

Clear dispersions of oil in water or water in oil are referred to as micro-emulsions. These appear homogeneous to the naked eye. These types of emulsions are also known as solubilized systems because macroscopically they seem to behave as true solutions but these micro-emulsions should not be confused with solutions formed by co-solvency.

Microemulsions can be prepared with emulsifying agents which give a local negative interfacial tension and form monomolecular interfacial films. Since these are clear preparations so becoming more popular day by day. Microemulsions are also free from some of the stability problems of emulsions.

Tests for Identification of Type of Emulsion

Since both the types (O/W) and (W/O) of emulsions are similar in appearance therefore it is very difficult to differentiate them with naked eye. They can be identified with the help of following tests but no one test gives correct results. Therefore the type of emulsion determined by one method should be confirmed by second method.

(a) Dilution Test

Take a few drops of emulsion in a test-tube and dilute it with 2-3 drops of water. If the water is distributed uniformly in the emulsion then the emulsion is O/W type but if water separates out as a layer then the emulsion is W/O type. Similarly on dilution with oil, the oil will distribute uniformly in W/O emulsion but separates out in O/W type emulsion.

(b) Conductivity Test

Water is a good conductor of electricity whereas oil is non-conductor of electricity. So conductivity test can be performed by dipping a pair of electrodes connected through a low voltage lamp, in the emulsion. On passing an electric current through the electrodes if the bulb glows, the emulsion is O/W type because water is in the continuous phase and current has passed through the water but if the bulb does not glow, the emulsion is W/O type because oil is in the continuous phase and the current has not passed through the oil which has failed to glow the bulb.

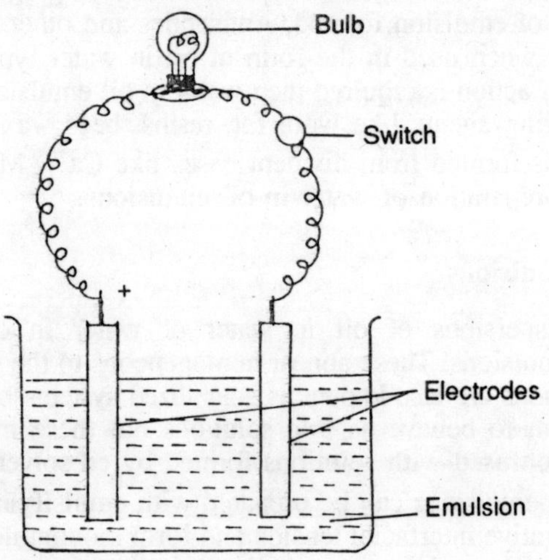

Fig. 8.1 Conductivity test.

(c) Dye-Solubility Test

Mix an oil soluble dye like scarlet red with an emulsion. Place a drop of it on a microscope slide and see under the microscope. If the continuous phase appears to be red, it is W/O emulsion but if scattered globules appears red and continuous phase colourless it is O/W emulsion. This test

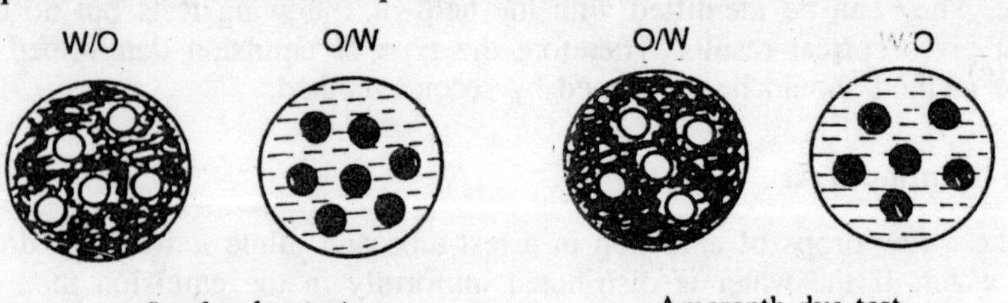

Scarlet dye test   Amaranth dye test

Fig. 8.2 Dye-solubility test.

can be repeated by using amaranth, a water soluble dye. If the continuous phase appears red it is O/W emulsion but if scattered globules appear red and continuous phase colourless it is W/O emulsion.

(d) $CoCl_2$ Filter Paper Test

When a filter paper impregnated with $CoCl_2$ and dried (blue) is dipped in an emulsion changes to pink, it indicates that emulsion is O/W type. This test may fail if emulsion is unstable or breaks in the presence of electrolytes.

(e) Fluorescence Test

When oils are exposed to U.V. rays they fluoresce, O/W emulsions exhibit spotty pattern and W/O emulsions fluoresce throughout the field. This method is not always applicable.

Out of these tests the first three are more reliable hence commonly used.

Emulsifying Agents

Emulsifying agents are also known as emulgents of emulsifiers. They reduce the interfacial tension between the two phases, i.e., aqueous phase and oily phase thus make them miscible with each other and form a stable emulsion. It is very difficult to select a proper emulsifying agent for the development of a stable emulsion.

No single emulsifying agent possesses all the properties required for the preparation of stable emulsion therefore sometimes it becomes necessary to use two or more than two emulsifying agents instead of one to get a product of desired qualities.

Classification of Emulsifying Agents

Emulsifying agents may be classified as follows :

1. Natural emulsifying agents from vegetable sources

(a) Acacia
(b) Tragacanth
(c) Agar
(d) Chondrus (Irish Moss)
(e) Pectin
(f) Starch.

2. Natural emulsifying agents from animal sources

(a) Gelatin
(b) Egg yolk
(c) Wool fat.

3. Semi-synthetic polysaccharides

(a) Methyl cellulose
(b) Sodium carboxymethyl cellulose.

4. Synthetic emulsifying agents

(a) Anionic
(b) Cationic
(c) Non-ionic.

5. Inorganic emulsifying agents

(a) Milk of magnesia
(b) Magnesium oxide
(c) Magnesium trisilicate
(d) Magnesium aluminium silicate
(e) Bentonite

6. Saponins

7. Alcohols

(a) Cholesterol
(b) Carbowaxes
(c) Lecithin.

1. Natural Emulsifying Agents from Vegetable Sources

The natural emulsifying agents obtained from vegetable sources are carbohydrates which include gums and mucilaginous substances. They are anionic in nature and produce O/W emulsions. Some of them act as true emulsifiers which are also known as primary emulsifying agents while others act as emulsion stabilizers also known as secondary emulsifying agents. They are capable of emulsifying a large number of substances but the resulting emulsions will have to be preserved by adding a suitable preservative because the carbohydrates act as very good medium for bacterial growth. The preservatives which can be added are alcohol, sodium benzoate, benzoic acid or a combination of methyl paraben and propyl paraben. These preservatives should be added carefully because high concentrations of alcohols and solutions of metallic salts may lead to cracking of emulsion.

(a) Acacia

Acacia is the best known emulsifying agent for the extemporaneous preparation of emulsions for internal use. Emulsions prepared with gum acacia are attractive in appearance, quite palatable and relatively stable. They are stable over a wide range of pH (2 to 10). These emulsions usually have low viscosity therefore creaming takes place quite rapidly which can be prevented by increasing the viscosity of the medium by incorporating tragacanth, agar or pectin along with acacia.

Emulsions prepared with acacia are susceptible to bacterial growth therefore they must be suitably preserved.

The ratio of powdered acacia usually taken for emulsification of fixed oils is 1 : 4 and for volatile oils is 1 : 2, that is 1 gram of acacia is sufficient to emulsify 4 ml of fixed oils and 2 ml of volatile oils. When mucilage of acacia is used, 1 gram is sufficient for 2 ml of oil.

(b) Tragacanth

Tragacanth alone is rarely used as an emulsifying agent because it does not reduce the interfacial tension and thus the oil globules are usually of large size. It produces very coarse and thick emulsions and sometimes viscosity increases to such an extent that pouring of the emulsion becomes a problem. A very stable emulsion is produced if both acacia and tragacanth are used as emulsifying agents for the preparation of an emulsion. Tragacanth will render the emulsion more viscous and thereby the rate of creaming will be reduced which is quite high in the case of acacia emulsions. The quantity of tragacanth required for this purpose is 1/10th of the amount of acacia used. The appearance and stability of the emulsions can be improved to a great extent by passing the finished product through a homogenizer.

(c) Agar

Agar is not a good emulsifying agent as it forms a very coarse and viscous emulsion. It is commonly used as a thickening agent along with acacia for the emulsification of mineral oils. Generally 2% mucilage of agar is prepared by dissolving it in boiling water and cooled to 45°C. Below this temperature it will form a gel which is not used in emulsions. The mucilage is incorporated in the primary emulsion in sufficient quantity to make 30 to 50 per cent of the final volume.

(d) Chondrus (Irish Moss)

Like agar, chondrus is also not used as a primary emulsifier but is used as a thickening agent. Generally it is used along with acacia for the emulsification of cod-liver oil and to mask the unpleasant odour and taste of the oil. A 3% solution is used to emulsify an equal volume of the oil.

(e) Pectin

Pectin is a purified complex carbohydrate obtained from the inner rind of citrus fruit and from the pulp of apple and guava. It acts as a emulsion stabilizer in acacia emulsions. If pectin alone is to be used as emulsifying agent a ratio of 0.1 gm per gram of acacia is sufficient for emulsification of the oil. A mucilage of pectin is first prepared before adding it to the preparation. To prevent the formation of lumps, pectin can be triturated with a small amount of alcohol, glycerol or syrup before the addition of water.

(f) Starch

Starch is rarely used as an emulsifying agent but the use of starch mucilage is restricted to preparations used as enemas.

2. Natural Emulsifying Agents from Animal Sources

(a) Gelatin

Gelatin is mainly used for the emulsification of liquid paraffin. 1% concentration forms the emulsions. Emulsions so formed are quite white and have an agreeable taste. However gelatin emulsions are prone to bacterial growth therefore a suitable preservative must be incorporated.

(b) Egg Yolk

Egg yolk itself is an emulsion because of the presence of lecithin and cholesterol which act as emulsifying agents. It is rarely used in industrial preparations because the emulsions are spoiled during transportation, therefore it is mainly used in extemporaneous preparations meant for internal use. It is generally used for the emulsification of fish liver oils. On an average 15 gram of egg yolk can be obtained from each egg which can emulsify about 120 ml of fixed oil and 60 ml of volatile oil. A suitable preservative must be added to emulsions prepared with egg yolk and further they must be stored in a refrigerator.

(c) Wool Fat (Anhydrous Lanolin)

Wool fat is generally used in emulsions meant for external application. It produces water in oil emulsions and can absorb about 50% of water but when mixed with other fatty substances it can emulsify several times its own weight of water and other hydroalcoholic liquids.

3. Semi-Synthetic Polysaccharides

(a) Methyl Cellulose

Methyl cellulose is a synthetic derivative of cellulose and is widely used in the pharmaceutical industry as suspending, thickening and emulsifying agent. It is available in different forms such as methyl cellulose 20, methyl cellulose 2500 and methyl cellulose 4500. The number indicates the average viscosity in centipoises of a 2 per cent aqueous solution. Methyl cellulose is commonly used for emulsification of mineral and vegetable oils but is less satisfactory for cod liver oil. Methyl cellulose is soluble in hot water therefore a special technique is used for quick preparation of mucilage. Emulsions prepared with methyl cellulose are very stable to pH changes and alcohol but may be precipitated in the presence of large amounts of electrolytes.

(b) ·'ium Carboxymethyl Cellulose

It is n ...d as a true emulsifier but is used as an emulsion stabilizer in the concentration of 0.5 to 1.0%. It is soluble in cold water as well as hot water.

4. Synthetic Emulsifying Agents

This group includes the surface active agents which are used as emulsifying agents. They are classified according to the ionic charge possessed by the molecules of the surfactant, e.g., anionic, cationic and non-ionic.

(a) Anionic

Various alkali soaps, metallic soaps, sulphated alcohols and sulphonates are used as emulsifying agents. They bear a negative charge on them. Soaps may be used as very good emulsifying agents but are mainly meant for external application. Soap emulsions have a high pH and are not stable at pH values less than 10. They are also precipitated by the addition of acids and electrolytes.

Among the sulphated alcohols, sodium lauryl sulphate is commonly used as emulsifying agent in topical preparations. It produces O/W emulsions.

Dioctyl sodium sulphosuccinate is an example of sulphonates which is widely used in the preparations of materials which are used to soften the stools. It is also used in topical preparations.

(b) Cationic

Cationic surface active agents bear positive charge on them. They are mainly used in the preparations meant for external use such as skin lotions and creams. They have marked bacterial properties therefore generally reserved for those preparations in which germicidal activity is required.

Quaternary ammonium compounds are the only group of cationic agents which are extensively used as emulsifying agents. These include benzalkonium chloride, benzethonium chloride, cetrimide, etc.

(c) Non-Ionic

The non-ionic surface active agents are widely used in the preparation of pharmaceutical emulsions because the emulsions prepared with non-ionic surfactants remain stable over a wide range of pH changes and are not affected by the addition of acids and electrolytes. The most commonly used non-ionic surface active agents are the glyceryl esters such as glyceryl monostearate, polyoxyethylene glycol esters and ethers, and sorbitan fatty acid esters such as sorbitan monopalmitate.

5. Inorganic Emulsifying Agents

Several inorganic substances such as milk of magnesia, magnesium oxide, magnesium trisilicate, magnesium aluminium silicate, bentonite, etc., are used in the preparation of pharmaceutical emulsions. Usually they produce O/W emulsions but bentonite may be used to prepare either O/W or W/O emulsions, depending on the order of mixing. 5% suspension of bentonite is used as an emulsifying agent. For the preparation of O/W emulsion, oil is added to the suspension of bentonite whereas for W/O emulsion the oil is placed in the container and then the bentonite suspension is added to the oil with rapid stirring.

6. Saponins

Saponins are rarely used as emulsifying agents. If specially prescribed then quillaia tincture and liquid extract may be used as emulsifying agents.

7. Alcohols

(a) Cholesterol

A number of high molecular weight alcohols are used in emulsion systems primarily for their stabilizing action. Cetyl alcohol, stearyl alcohol, cholesterol and glyceryl monostearate may be included in this group. They are rarely used as single emulsifying agent therefore other emulsifying agents must be included in the emulsion system to achieve good results.

(b) Carbowaxes

Carbowaxes act as non-ionic emulsifying agents and mainly used in the preparation of ointments and creams. Their molecular weight varies from 200 to 1000. Carbowax 200 to 700 are viscous, light coloured hygroscopic liquids whereas carbowax with molecular weight 1000 and above are wax like solids. A product with desired consistency can be produced by using suitable carbowaxes.

(c) Lecithins

Lecithin forms W/O emulsions but is rarely used as emulsifying agent because it darkens in colour when exposed to light and gets easily oxidised.

Hydrophile-Lipophile Balance (HLB)

Griffin (1954) devised a useful system of classification of non-ionic surfactants related to their behavior and their solubility in water. Thus providing a particular type of emulsion. The numerical values, called the Hydrophile-Lipophile Balance (HLB), denote the relative affinity for oil and water. Oil soluble materials have low values while water-soluble materials have high values. Commonly used emulsifying agents have HLB values ranging form 1 to 40. Emulsifying agents with high HLB values i.e. 7 to 20 produce O/W emulsions (hydrophilic) and those with low HLB values i.e. 3 to 6 produce W/O emulsion (lipophilic)

The following table indicates the HLB values and applications of emulsifying agents.

HLB values of emulsifying agents and their applications

S. No.	Name of the emulsifying agent	HLB value	Applications	Type of emulsion
1.	Acacia	8.0	Emulsifying agent	O/W
2.	Glyceryl monostearate	3.8	Emulsifying agent	W/O
3.	Sorbitan monooleate	4.3	Emulsifying agent	W/O
4.	Sorbitan mono-stearate	4.7	Emulsifying agent	W/O
5.	Polysorbate 20	16.7	Solubilising agent	—
6.	Polysorbate 60	14.9	Detergent	—
7.	Polysorbate 80	15.0	Solubilising agent	—
8.	Sodium lauryl sulphate	40.0	Emulsifying agent	O/W
9.	Sodium oleate	18.0	Solubilising agent	—
10.	Tragacanth	13.2	Emulsifying agent	O/W
11.	Triethanolamine oleate	12.0	Emulsifying agent	O/W

Choice of Emulsifying Agents

To get an emulsion of required properties, the emulsifying agent selected must have the following qualities:

1. It should be capable of reducing the interfacial tension between the two immiscible liquids.
2. It should be capable of keeping the globules of dispersed liquid distributed indefinitely throughout the dispersion medium.
3. It should be non-toxic.
4. The odour and taste should be compatible with the preparation.
5. It should be chemically compatible with other ingredients of the preparation.
6. It should be able to produce and maintain the required consistency of the preparation.

Preparation of Emulsions

For small-scale work emulsions can be prepared by the following methods :

(a) Dry gum method
(b) Wet gum method
(c) Bottle method.

In dry gum method the oil is first triturated with gum and then water is added to make a primary emulsion whereas in wet gum method the gum is first triturated with water to form a mucilage and then oil is incorporated in small quantities with constant trituration to form a primary emulsion.

For extemporaneous compounding of emulsions by dry gum method and wet gum method the most efficient apparatus used is mortar and pestle. The mortar should be flat bottomed and rough on the inner surface so as to produce fine particles of the dispersed globules. Glass mortars should not be used because of their smooth surface.

Table given below shows the proportions of oil, water and gum acacia required for fixed oils and volatile oils for the preparation of primary emulsion.

Proportion of	*Oil*	:	*Water*	:	*Gum*
Fixed oils	4	:	2	:	1
Volatile oils	4	:	4	:	2

The most commonly used fixed oils and volatile oils are :

Fixed Oils

Castor oil, cod liver oil, shark liver oil, olive oil, almond oil and liquid paraffin (mineral oil).

Volatile Oils

Turpentine oil, sandal wood oil, cinnamon oil and peppermint oil.

(a) Dry Gum Method

This method is also known as 4 : 2 : 1 method because these figures represent the proportions of oil, water and gum acacia required for the preparation of primary emulsion. That is, for example, if there are 40 ml of fixed oil to be emulsified then 10 gm of gum acacia and 20 ml of water or vehicle will be required for preparing the primary emulsion.

Measure the given quantity of oil with a clean and dry measure and transfer it to a dry mortar. To this add the calculated quantity of acacia and triturate rapidly so as to form a uniform mixture. Then add the required quantity of water for primary emulsion and triturate rapidly without ceasing till a clicking sound is produced and the product becomes white or nearly white. At this stage the emulsion is known as primary emulsion. Then add more of water to produce the required volume. If any soluble ingredient is also to be incorporated, that must be dissolved in the second portion of water to be added after making the primary emulsion and to produce the final volume.

(b) Wet Gum Method

The proportions of oil, water and gum are same as for dry gum method. In this method the calculated quantity of gum is triturated with water to form a mucilage. Then the given amount of oil is incorporated in small portions with rapid trituration until a clicking sound is produced and the product becomes white or nearly so. When the primary emulsion is formed, the trituration in continued for few minutes more and then more of water is incorporated in successive small portions to produce the required volume.

(c) Bottle Method

Bottle method is used for the preparation of emulsions of volatile and other non-viscous oils. The emulsions can be prepared by both the dry gum and wet gum methods. Because of low viscosity the volatile oils require greater amount of gum for emulsification therefore the proportions for oil, water and gum for primary emulsion are 4 : 4 : 2.

In this method the oil is put in a large bottle and then the powdered dry gum is added. The bottle is shaken vigorously until the oil and gum are mixed thoroughly. Then the calculated amount of water is added all at once and the mixture is shaken vigorously until primary emulsion is formed. More of water is added in small portions with constant agitation after each addition, to produce the final volume.

Other Methods

Various homogenisers and blenders are used for preparing emulsions. Q.P. homogeniser is the most widely used hand homogeniser for extemporaneous preparations. A coarse emulsion is prepared in a mortar which is then transfered to the hand homogeniser wherein the emulsion is forced to pass through a narrow aperture under pressure and thereby the particle size of the globules is reduced. The emulsion may be passed through the homogeniser several times until a satisfactory product is formed. The reduction of particle size of globules increases with the speed of pumping.

Stability of Emulsions

Stability of emulsion means that a formulated emulsion should retain its original characters, i.e., regarding the size of globules and their uniform distribution throughout the continuous phase. Emulsions should be chemically stable and they should not allow any bacterial growth to take place.

In the present discussion only the physical stability will be discussed

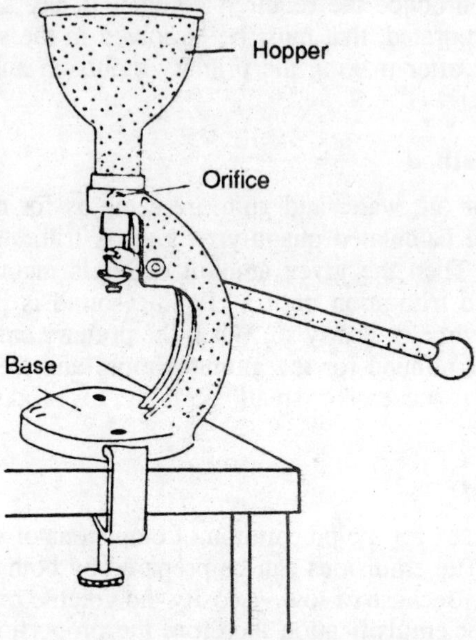

Fig. 8.3 Q.P. emulsifier.

in detail. The three major changes associated with physical stability are as follows :

1. Upward or downward movement of dispersed globules in the continuous phase referred to as creaming or sedimentation of emulsions.
2. Aggregation of the dispersed globules forming a separate phase referred to as cracking of emulsions.
3. Phase inversion.

Creaming and Sedimentation

In creaming the dispersed globules move upward and form a thick layer at the surface of the emulsion whereas in sedimentation the dispersed globules move downward towards the bottom and form a layer over there. A good example of creaming is when milk is set aside for a few hours, a thick layer of cream forms at the surface. Creaming is a temporary phase because it can be re-distributed by mild shaking or stirring to get a homogenous product. At the same time creaming is undesirable because a badly creamed emulsion may lead to cracking with complete separation of the two phases. There are many factors which lead to creaming of emulsions but the chief factor is the rising of dispersed globules to the surface of the emulsion. The rate at which the globules will rise to the surface or the rate of creaming is governed by Stoke's law, which may be expressed as follows :

$$V = \frac{2r^2 (d_1 - d_2) g}{9\eta}$$

where V = rate of creaming

r = radius of globules

d_1 = density of dispersed phase

d_2 = density of continuous phase

g = gravitational constant

η = viscosity of the dispersion medium.

It is evident from the equation that the rate of creaming depends upon the radius of globules, the difference between the densities of the dispersed phase and continuous phase and the viscosity of the dispersion medium. Larger the size of the globules more will be creaming and smaller the size of the globules lesser will be creaming because small globules will rise less quickly than large globules. Therefore creaming can be reduced by reducing the size of globules by passing the emulsion through a homogeniser.

The rate of creaming depends upon the difference between the densities of dispersed phase and continuous phase. Greater the difference more will be creaming. Therefore this difference can be reduced but this is rarely possible in practice because it is therapeutically undesirable.

The rate of creaming is inversely proportional to the viscosity of the dispersion medium, therefore this is the most suitable approach for preparing a stable emulsion. The viscosity of the emulsion can be increased, but too high a viscosity is undesirable because it may become difficult to redisperse the materials which have settled and pouring of the too viscous product from its container may be a problem.

The high temperature reduces viscosity which encourages creaming, therefore emulsions should be stored in a cool place. Freezing should be avoided which may lead to cracking.

Cracking

In cracking the coalescence of the dispersed globules takes place and two separate layers of the dispersed phase and continuous phase are formed which are difficult to redisperse by shaking or stirring to get the original product. Hence cracking is more serious in comparison to creaming. Cracking may take place due to following reasons :

(a) By addition of emulsifying agent of opposite type

As discussed earlier soaps of monovalent metals produce O/W type emulsions whereas soaps of divalent metals produce W/O type emulsions. But the addition of monovalent soap to an emulsion prepared with divalent soap or vice versa will lead to instability and cracking of emulsion.

(b) By decomposition or precipitation of emulsifying agents

The addition of an acid to an alkali soap emulsion, e.g., turpentine liniment, leads to decomposition of the emulsifying agent with the liberation of fatty acid and alkali salt of the added acid, neither of which has emulsifying properties thus causing cracking.

The addition of sodium chloride and certain other electrolytes to sodium soap or potassium soap emulsions leads to the precipitation of emulsifying agent thus causing cracking.

(c) By addition of a common solvent

The addition of a solvent to an emulsion, which is either miscible with or can dissolve the dispersed phase, the emulsifying agent and the continuous phase leads to the formation of one phase system or clear solution thus destroying the emulsion. For example, when alcohol is added to turpentine oil liniment it forms a clear solution because turpentine oil, soft soap and water gets dissolved in alcohol.

(d) By micro-organisms

The emulsions which are stored for a long time may develop bacterial and mold growth which may destroy the emulsifying agent and cause cracking. Therefore the emulsions which are not meant for immediate use must be suitably preserved.

(e) By high temperature

When emulsions are stored for a long time an increase in temperature may reduce viscosity of the emulsion and encourage creaming.

(f) By creaming

A badly creamed emulsion is more liable to crack than a homogeneous emulsion therefore steps should be taken to retard creaming as for as possible.

Phase Inversion

In phase inversion the oil in water type emulsion changes into water in oil type and vice versa. It is a physical instability. It may be brought about by the addition of an electrolyte or by changing the phase-volume ratio or by temperature changes, etc. Phase inversion can be minimised by using the proper emulsifying agent in adequate concentration, keeping the concentration of dispersed phase between 30 to 60 per cent (higher concentration may lead to phase inversion) and by storing the emulsion in a cool place.

Instability of Emulsions

Instability of an emulsion is not due to only creaming, cracking or phase inversion but it may be due to other reasons also. Instability has been observed when the medicament is suspended in an emulsion. For example, in the case of liquid paraffin and phenolphthalein emulsion the phenolphthalein should be very finely dispersed throughout the emulsion otherwise it will settle down which will be very difficult to redisperse on shaking.

Occasionally emulsions are intentionally made with an inherent instability. An O/W barrier cream may be used which liberates a film of oil when applied to the skin. Sometimes emulsion breaking is an essential part of a manufacturing process such as the separation of wool fat from wool scouring waste.

Preservation of Emulsions

Since emulsions are prepared by using emulsifying agents such as carbohydrates, proteins, sterols and non-ionic surfactants which lead to the growth of bacteria, fungi, molds and yeasts, specially in the presence of water. The contamination of emulsions by these micro-organisms may cause unpleasant odour, taste and discolouration. The eating up of the emulsifying agent by the microorganisms will lead to changes in consistency and ultimately may cause cracking. Even if the emulsion does not crack it will become unfit for consumption. Other factors affecting growth of microorganisms in emulsions include :

(a) Deionised water and purified water if not stored properly after collection.
(b) Carelessly cleaned equipment.
(c) Type of container and closure used.
(d) The ratio of oil and water and the type of emulsion.
(e) pH of the preparation.

The above mentioned factors can be minimized to a great extent by :

(a) Using ingredients of high quality.
(b) Using boiling water to destroy the microorganisms.
(c) Using thoroughly cleaned equipment and paying particular attention to hidden parts of the equipment which are generally a major source of contamination.
(d) Using containers and closures of high quality and closures should fit well in the containers.
(e) Maintaining the prescribed ratio of oil and water.
(f) Maintaining the prescribed pH of the preparation.

The above mentioned precautions will not completely exclude the contamination therefore a suitable preservative will have to be included in the emulsion. The preservative used should have the following qualities :

1. It should be non-toxic.
2. It should be water soluble.
3. It should be effective in low concentrations.
4. It should be compatible with other ingredients of the preparation.

5. It should be effective against wide range of microorganisms.
6. It should be free from odour and taste.

Some of the commonly used preservatives in emulsions include benzoic acid, p-hydroxybenzoic acid, sodium benzoate, esters of p-hydroxybenzoic acid, chloroform, chlorocresol, and quaternary ammonium compounds, etc. Generally combinations of preservatives are used because they increase the preservation action by their synergistic effect.

Benzoic acid is commonly used for oral preparations the action of which is enhanced by the addition of chloroform as in liquid paraffin emulsions. Esters of p-hydroxybenzoic acid are popular preservatives which are used for oral as well as for external preparations. They are stable, inert, non-toxic, odourless and tasteless. They are effective against molds and yeasts, but less effective against bacteria. Sometimes the drug itself has a preservative action as in the cetrimide cream but in other preparations chlorocresol is the most suitable preservative.

Preservation from Oxidation

Substances like fats and oils obtained from vegetable and animal sources and certain emulsifying agents such as wool fat, wool alcohol and carbomer undergo oxidation by atmospheric oxygen which should be prevented by adding antioxidants. Sometimes oxidation occurs due to enzymes produced by microorganisms which should be prevented by adding suitable antimicrobial preservative.

Rx

Castor oil	8 ml
Water ad	30 ml

Fiat : Emulsio.
Signa : More dicto sumenda.
Type : O/w type emulsion for internal use.

Theory

Castor oil is a fixed oil and is not miscible with water. To make it miscible a third substance known as emulsifying agent in the ratio of 4 : 2 : 1, i.e., oil : water : gum will be used for the preparation of primary emulsion. Gum acacia will be used as emulsifying agent because emulsions prepared with gum acacia remain stable for sufficiently long time.

Formula for primary emulsion :

Oil	:	*Water*	:	*Gum*
4	:	2	:	1
8 ml	:	4 ml	:	2 gm

Procedure

Wet gum method

Thoroughly clean and dry a pestle and mortar. Weigh out 2 gm gum acacia and transfer it to the mortar. Measure 4 ml water and triturate it with gum so as to form a mucilage. To this add 8 ml castor oil in small quantities at a time with thorough trituration after each addition. Triturate briskly without ceasing until a clicking sound is produced and the product becomes white or nearly white. At this stage the emulsion is known as primary emulsion. Add about 10 ml more of vehicle in small quantities at a time with constant trituration so as to get a homogenous product.

Transfer the emulsion to a measure, add more of vehicle to produce the final volume 30 ml, stir thoroughly so as to form a uniform emulsion. Transfer the preparation to a bottle, cork, polish the bottle to remove finger prints, label and dispense. Attach the secondary label "Shake well before use.".

Rx

Calciferol solution	0.15	ml
Glycerin	0.3	ml
Water ad	5.0	ml

Fiat emulsio. Mitte 50 ml.

Signa : 5 ml to be taken daily.

Type : O/w type emulsion for internal use containing a small volume of oily substance.

Theory

In this prescription the quantity of calciferol solution (an oily liquid) prescribed is very small, i.e., about 3 percent. Generally speaking, emulsions containing appreciably less than 20% of oily liquid and prepared with the usual proportion of gum acacia, become unstable and readily cream. Therefore to prevent creaming, a bland of fixed oil (e.g., arachis, almond or olive) should be added to raise the total quantity of oily liquid to approximately 20%.

The substances which are prescribed in this way and require previous dilution with a fixed oil before emulsification include calciferol solution, concentrated solution of vitamin A, concentrated solution of vitamin A and D, concentrated solution of vitamin D, halibut liver oil and bromoform.

Formula for 50 ml primary emulsion :

Calciferol solution	1.5 ml
Olive oil	8.5 ml
Powdered acacia	2.5 gm
Water	5.0 ml

Procedure

Dry gum method

Take the calculated quantities of calciferol solution and olive oil in a dry mortar, add acacia powder and mix thoroughly. To this add measured amount of water, little at a time with continuous trituration until a white product is obtained and a clicking sound is produced. At this stage the emulsion is known as primary emulsion.

To the primary emulsion add glycerin with trituration. Incorporate more vehicle to dilute the emulsion. Transfer to a measure, rinse the mortar with small quantity of vehicle, add the rinsings to the measure. Incorporate more of vehicle to produce the required volume. Transfer the preparation to a bottle cork, polish, label and dispense. Attach "Shake the bottle before use." label.

Rx

Liquid paraffin	60.0 ml
Phenolphthalein	2.0 gm
Agar	1.5 gm
Acacia	15.0 gm
Syrup	15.0 ml
Cinnamon water to	180.0 ml

Make an emulsion.

Sig : One tablespoonful to be taken twice a day.

Type : O/w type emulsion containing oil and water insoluble substance, i.e., phenolphthalein.

Theory

Phenolphthalein is insoluble in liquid paraffin and water therefore it will have to be finely powdered if already not in fine powder, then mix with acacia before adding liquid paraffin and water to get primary emulsion. The final emulsion will have to be passed through a homogeniser to further reduce the particle size to get a stable and whiter emulsion because the ordinarily prepared liquid paraffin emulsions are very coarse in nature.

Formula for primary emulsion :

Liquid paraffin	60 ml
Phenolphthalein	2 gm
Acacia	15 gm
Cinnamon water	30 ml

Procedure

Finely powder phenolphthalein in a mortar. Mix it with acacia, add liquid paraffin and triturate. Incorporate cinnamon water required for primary emulsion, little at a time with constant trituration until a clicking sound is produced and a white product is formed. This will constitute the primary emulsion, the volume of which will be approximately 107 ml.

Separately in a tared dish dissolve agar in about 60 ml water by gentle heat; while hot adjust the volume to 60 ml because during heating small quantity of water will evaporate, therefore the volume is adjusted. Add syrup and cinnamon water, stir so as to get a uniform mass.

Gradually add the hot agar solution to the warm primary emulsion with constant trituration until uniform. Pass the product through a homogeniser in order to further reduce the particle size of the oil globules to get a stable and whiter product. Pass sufficient vehicle through the homogeniser to produce the required volume. Transfer to a bottle, label and dispense. Attach the secondary label, "Shake the bottle before use.".

Uses

This preparation is used as purgative.

1. Phenolphthalein is an irritant purgative which is usually given at night to act in the morning. It is administered alone or along with other purgatives such as liquid paraffin which enhances its action.
2. Acacia acts as an emulsifying agent but because of low viscosity a stable emulsion is not produced. To increase the viscosity agar is used as secondary emulsifying agent. Only a very small proportion of agar in solution can be included in an emulsion. More than 1% agar will produce a solid or semi-solid preparation, so agar must be used in proper proportion only along with primary emulsifier.
3. Syrup acts as a sweetening agent and cinnamon water as flavouring agent.

Marketed Emulsions

1. Agrol emulsion (Warner-Hindustan Division, Bombay - 400072).

   Each 30 ml contains :

Liquid paraffin	9.54	ml
Phenolphthalein	400	mg
Agar	60	mg

   Emulsifying agents and excipients to 30 ml in aqueous base containing glycerin and sorbitol solution.

2. Cremaffin liquid (Boots Pharmaceuticals Ltd., Bombay - 400038).

   Each 15 ml contains :

Milk of magnesia	11.25	ml
Liquid paraffin	3.75	ml

3. Laxol-P liquid (Medochem Labs Pvt. Ltd., Delhi - 110032).

   Each 30 ml contains :

Paraffin	9.54	ml
Phenolphthalein	400	mg
Agar-agar	60	mg

4. Magafin emulsion (Reliable Laboratories Pvt. Ltd., New Delhi 110020).

Each 15 ml contains :

Milk of magnesia	11.25	ml
Liquid paraffin	3.75	ml
Phenolphthalein	50.0	mg

5. Phenolax liquid (Rays Labs Pvt. Ltd., Calcutta - 700007).

Each 5 ml contains :

Liquid paraffin	1.25	ml
Phenolphthalein	17.0	mg
Mag. hydroxide	100.0	mg

Revision Questions

I. Very short answer type questions

(A) Define the following :

(a) Emulsion
(b) Emulsifying agent/emulgents
(c) Microemulsions
(d) Creaming of emulsions
(e) Cracking of emulsions
(f) HLB

(B)

(a) Explain why emulsions are prepared or write advantage of emulsions
(b) What is Stokes' Law? Write the equation of Stokes' Law.
(c) Give a list of emulsifying agents obtained from vegetable sources.
(d) Why all most all the emulsions appear milky white.

(e) Write the proportion of oil, water and gum used in the preparation of primary emulsion for
   - (i) Fixed oil
   - (ii) Volatile oil
   - (iii) Mineral oil

(f) Give example of
   - (a) Fixed oils
   - (b) Volatile oils
   - (c) Mineral oil

(C) Fill in the blanks

(i) When two immiscible liquids are made miscible with each other in the presence of ...... it is known as ......

(ii) Emulsifying agents reduce ...... between two phases.

(iii) In o/w type emulsion, ... is in disperse phase where as ...... is in continuous phase.

(iv) O/W type emulsions are generally meant for ...... use where as W/O type emulsions are generally meant for ...... use.

(v) Soaps formed from ...... are used for preparing o/w type emulsions where as soaps formed from ...... are used for preparing w/o emulsions.

(vi) The rate of creaming is governed by a law known as ......

(vii) In an emulsion complete separation of two phases is known as ......

(viii) When w/o type emulsion changes into o/w type and vice versa, this phenomena is known as ......

II. Short answer type questions

Write short notes on :

(i) Tests for the identification of type of emulsion.

(ii) Advantages of emulsions

(iii) Qualities of an emulsifying agent.

(iv) Creaming of emulsion

(v) Cracking of emulsion

(vi) Micro-emulsions

(vii) Q.P. homogenizer

(viii) Preservation of emulsions

(ix) Stokes' law

(x) Dry gum method

III. Long answer type questions

1. What is an emulsion? Discuss different types of emulsions and various tests to identify them.
2. What are emulgents? Classify the emulgents and explain briefly the different emulgents used in the formulation of emulsions.
3. Enumerate different types of emulsifying agents. Give suitable examples of emulsifying agents which will produce :
   (a) O/W type emulsions
   (b) W/O type emulsions
   (c) Emulsions meant for internal use
   (d) Emulsions meant for external use
4. (a) Discuss briefly the object of combining acacia and tragacanth in the formulation of emulsions. What proportion of acacia is used in emulsions containing fixed oils/volatile oils and when both type of oils are present in one formulation.
   (b) Describe the methods by which the type of an emulsion can be determined.
5. Describe different methods of preparation of emulsions. Discuss advantages of one method over the other.
6. What do you understand by the terms 'creaming' and 'cracking' of emulsions? Discuss the factors which lead to creaming and cracking of emulsions.
7. Discuss the factors which govern the stability of emulsions and explain how the creaming in emulsions may be minimized.
8. What are emulsions? Discuss in brief the various methods used for the preparation of emulsions.
9. Differentiate between the following :
   (a) O/W and W/O emulsions
   (b) Creaming and cracking
   (c) Dry gum method and wet gum method
   (d) Emulsion and suspension.

3. What are the different methods of preparing emulsions? Discuss the significance of Stokes' law in stability of emulsions.
4. Give at least three examples of marketed emulsions.

Answers

I (C)

(i) Emulsifying agent, emulsion
(ii) Interfacial tension
(iii) Oil, water

(iv) Internal, external
(v) Monovalent basis, divalent bases
(vi) Stokes' law
(vii) Cracking
(viii) Phase inversion

9

Semisolid Dosage Forms

OINTMENTS, CREAMS, PASTES AND JELLIES

Ointments

Ointments are the soft semisolid preparations meant for external application to the skin or mucous membrane. They usually contain a medicament or medicaments dissolves, suspended or emulsified in the base. Ointments are used for their emollient and protective action to the skin. They may also be used as vehicles or bases for the topical application of medicinal substances.

The absorption of medicaments by the tissues from the ointment or other semisolid preparations applied to the skin depends upon a number of factors, e.g., properties of the drugs incorporated, properties of the bases used in the formulation, condition of the patient's skin, site of application, duration of application and degree of friction used in the application of the preparation.

Creams

Creams are thought of as ointments but usually contain a water soluble base due to which they can be easily removed from the skin. They are of a softer consistency and have a lighter body than true ointment. When applied to the skin, leave no visible evidence of their presence on the skin.

Pastes

Pastes are the semisolid preparations meant for application to the skin. They differ from ointments that they generally contain a large amount of finely powdered solids such as starch, zinc oxide, calcium carbonate, etc. Due to the presence of these substances they usually become quite thick and stiff than the ointments but are less greasy than ointments.

Since pastes are stiff they do not melt at ordinary temperature thus forming and holding a protective coating over the areas to which they are applied. They can be applied to the affected part with the help of a spatula or they may be spread on any of the dressing material and then applied. They are not removed for quite a long time. The pastes are not suitable for application to the hair because they are very difficult to remove from there.

Jellies

Jellies are thin transparent or translucent, non-greasy preparations meant for external application to the skin. They are similar to mucilages because they are prepared by using gums but they differ from mucilages in having jelly like consistency. They are used chiefly on mucous membranes for their lubricating, antiseptic or spermicidal purposes. Jellies are also used for lubricating surgical gloves, catheters and rectal thermometers. Vaginal jellies and contraceptive jellies are also commonly used.

Since jellies contain carbohydrates and lot of water as base therefore they are prone to microbial growth so they must be suitably preserved. The commonly used gelling agents for the preparation of jellies are tragacanth, sodium alginate, starch, pectin, gelatin, methyl cellulose, carbomer, polyvinyl alcohols, etc.

Characteristics of an Ideal Ointment

1. It should be chemically and physically stable.
2. It should be smooth and free from grittyness.
3. It should melt or soften at body temperature and be easily applied.
4. The base should be non-irritating and should have no therapeutic action.
5. The medicament should be finely divided and uniformly distributed throughout the base.

Classification of Ointments

Ointments may be classified as follows :

1. According to their therapeutic properties based on penetration.
2. According to their therapeutic uses.

1. Ointments classified according to their therapeutic properties based on penetration are as follows :

(a) Epidermic
(b) Endodermic
(c) Diadermic.

(a) Epidermic Ointments

These ointments are intended to produce their action on the surface of the skin and produce local effect. They are not absorbed. These types of ointments act as protectives, antiseptics, local anti-infectives and parasiticides.

(b) Endo-dermic Ointments

These ointments are intended to release medicaments that penetrate into the skin. They are partially absorbed and act as emollients, stimulants and local irritants.

(c) Diadermic Ointments

These ointments are intended to release the medicaments that pass through the skin and produce systemic effects.

2. According to therapeutic uses the ointments are classified as follows :

(i) Antieczematous Ointments

These ointments are used to remove oozing and excretion from vesicles on the skin. The drugs used are hydrocortisones, coal tar, ichthammol and salicylic acid.

(ii) Antibiotic Ointments

These ointments are used to kill the micro-organisms. The agents used are bacitracin, chlortetracycline, neomycin, quaternary ammonium compounds, etc.

(iii) Antifungal Ointments

These ointments are used to inhibit or kill the fungi. The agents used are benzoic acid, salicylic acid, nystatin, etc.

(iv) Anti-inflammatory Ointments

These ointments are used to relieve inflammatory, allergic and pruritic conditions of the skin. Generally betamethasone valerate, hydrocortisone and its acetate, triamcinolone acetonide, etc., are used for this purpose.

(v) Antipruritic Ointments

These ointments are used to relieve itching. Drugs for this purpose include benzocaine and coal tar.

(vi) Astringent Ointments

These ointments cause contraction of the skin and decrease discharges. Examples of astringents include calamine, zinc oxide, aluminium acetate and subacetate, acetic acid and tannic acid.

(vii) Counter-irritant Ointments

These ointments are applied locally to irritate the intact skin thus reducing or relieving another irritation or deep seated pain. The drugs used are capsicum oleoresin, iodine, methyl salicylate.

(viii) Ointments used for dandruff treatment

Drugs include salicylic acid and cetrimide.

(ix) Emollients

These are the preparations which are used to soften the skin. The agents include soft paraffins, cold cream and water in oil emulsion bases.

(x) Keratolytic and Keratoplastic Ointments

Keratolytic ointments are used to remove or soften the horney layer of the skin. The substances include resorcinol, salicylic acid and sulphur. Keratoplastic substances tend to increase the thickness of horney layer. The examples include coal tar.

(xi) Parasiticide Ointments

These ointments destroy or inhibit living infestations such as lice and ticks. Substances incorporated into parasiticide ointments, creams or lotions include benzyl benzoate, gamma-benzene hexachloride, sulphur, etc.

(xii) Protectant Ointments

These ointments protect the skin from moisture, air, sun rays or other substances such as soaps or chemicals. The agents which are used in protectant ointments include silicones, petrolatum, titanium dioxide, calamine, zinc oxide, etc.

Ointment Bases

The ointment base is that substance or part of an ointment which serves as a carrier or vehicle for the medicament. An ideal ointment base should be inert, stable, smooth, compatible with the skin, non-irritating and should release the incorporated medicament readily. Since there is no single ointment base available which possesses all these qualities, therefore it becomes necessary to use more than one ointment base in the preparation of ointments.

Classification of Ointment Bases

The ointment bases are classified as follows :

1. Oleaginous bases
2. Absorption bases
3. Emulsion bases
4. Water soluble bases.

1. Oleaginous Bases

These bases consist of water insoluble hydrophobic oils and fats. The most important are the hydrocarbons, i.e., mineral oils, petrolatums and paraffins. The animal fat includes lard. The combination of these materials can produce a product having desired melting point and viscosity. The oleaginous bases are decreasing in favour due to the reasons described below :

1. They are greasy.
2. They are difficult to remove both from skin and clothings.
3. The release of medicament is not certain.
4. If some animal fat is included it may get rancid.
5. Fatty mixture bases prevent drainage on oozing areas and also prevent evaporation of cutaneous secretions including perspiration. The water retention increases the heat in the particular areas.

Hydrocarbon Bases

(i) Petrolatum (Soft Paraffin)

It is a purified mixture of semisolid hydrocarbons obtained from petroleum. There are two varieties of soft paraffins, one is yellow soft paraffin and the other is white soft paraffin. Yellow soft paraffin is a pale yellow to yellow translucent soft mass, free or almost free from odour and taste. It has a melting point of 38°C to 56°C.

White soft paraffin is obtained by bleaching yellow soft paraffin. It is a white translucent tasteless mass and is odourless when rubbed on the skin. It has a melting point of 38°C to 56°C. White soft paraffin is used when the medicament is white or colourless.

Both yellow and white soft paraffins are used and have no noticeable action on the skin and are not absorbed. Thus they are suitable for epidermal type of preparations. Because of hydrophobic nature, aqueous liquids cannot be mixed with it but sometimes wool fat and waxes are included to incorporate aqueous liquids in it.

(ii) Hard Paraffin

It is a purified mixture of solid hydrocarbons obtained by distillation from petroleum or shale oil. It is a colourless or white translucent, odourless, tasteless mass and is used to harden or stiffen the ointment bases.

(iii) Liquid Paraffin

It is also known as liquid petrolatum or white mineral oil. It consists of a mixture of liquid hydrocarbons and may be obtained from petroleum by distillation. Liquid paraffin varies in composition according to the source of the petroleum. It is a colourless, transparent, tasteless and odourless oily liquid. It is insoluble in water and alcohol but soluble in ether and chloroform.

It is used along with hard paraffin and soft paraffin to get a desired consistency of the ointment. It is also used to levigate the substances insoluble in it.

2. Absorption Bases

The term absorption is used to denote the hydrophilic characters of the base. These are generally anhydrous bases which can absorb a large amount of water but still retain their ointment like consistency. The following are some of the absorption bases used.

(i) Wool Fat

It is also known as anhydrous lanolin. It is the purified anhydrous fat like substance obtained from the wool of sheep. It is practically insoluble in water but can absorb about 50% of its weight of water. Therefore it is used in ointments where the proportion of water or aqueous liquids to be incorporated in hydrocarbon base is too large. Due to its sticky nature it is not used alone but is used along with other bases in the preparation of a number of ointments.

(ii) Hydrous Wool Fat

It is also known as lanolin. It is the purified fat like substance obtained from wool of sheep. It is a yellowish white ointment like mass with characteristic odour. It is insoluble in water but soluble in ether and chloroform.

Hydrous wool fat is a mixture of 70% w/w wool fat and 30% w/w purified water. It is a water in oil emulsion. Aqueous liquids can be emulsified with it.

(iii) Wool Alcohol

It is obtained from wool fat by treating it with alkali and separating the fraction containing cholesterol and other alcohols. It contains not less than 30% of cholesterol. It is used as an emulsifying agent for the preparation of water in oil emulsions and is used to absorb water in ointment bases. It is also used to improve the texture, stability and emollient properties of oil in water emulsions.

(iv) Bees Wax

It is purified wax obtained from the honeycomb of bees. It is of two types : (a) yellow bees wax and (b) white bees wax obtained by bleaching and purifying the yellow bees wax. Bees wax is used as a stiffening agent in pastes, ointments and other preparations.

(v) Cholesterol

It is widely distributed in animal organisms. Wool fat is also used as a source of cholesterol. It is used to increase the incorporation of aqueous substances in oils and fats.

Advantages of Absorption Bases

(i) They are compatible with majority of medicaments.
(ii) They are relatively heat stable.

(iii) These bases may be used in their anhydrous form or in emulsified form.

(iv) They can absorb a large quantity of water or aqueous substances.

Disadvantages

These bases possess the undesirable property of greasiness but they can be more easily removed from the skin as compared to the oily bases.

3. Emulsion Bases

Emulsion bases are semisolid emulsions having cream like consistency. These are of two types : oil in water or water in oil emulsions. Some additional amount of water can be incorporated in both the types and still retain soft cream like consistency. The oil in water type emulsion bases are more popular because they can be easily removed from the skin or clothings by washing with water. The water in oil emulsion bases are greasy and sticky, therefore they are difficult to remove from the body and clothings. Examples of emulsion bases include hydrophilic ointment, rose water ointment and vanishing creams.

4. Water Soluble Bases

Water soluble bases contain only the water soluble ingredients and not the fats or other greasy substances that is why sometimes they are known as greaseless bases. They differ from emulsion bases that the latter contain water soluble and water insoluble components. Since these bases do not contain any fats or oils, they can be easily washed with water from the skin and clothings.

Water soluble bases consist of water soluble ingredients such as polyethylene glycol polymers which are popularly known as carbowaxes. Carbowaxes are water soluble, non-volatile, inert substances. They do not hydrolyse and do not support the bacterial or mold growth. The release of medicament is rapid. Depending upon the molecular weight carbowaxes are available in different consistencies, i.e., liquids, semisolids and solids. Their molecular weight varies from 200 to 8000. As the molecular weight goes on increasing the solidity and whiteness also goes on increasing. Carbowax 200, 300, 400 are viscous liquids; carbowax 1500 is soft greasy semisolid having the consistency like that of petrolatum; carbowax 1540, 3000, 4000 to 6000 are waxy solids. A blend of different carbowaxes is used to get an ointment of desired consistency.

Certain other substances which are used as water soluble bases include tragacanth, gelatin, pectin, silica gel, sodium alginate, cellulose derivatives, magnesium-aluminium silicate and bentonite. In the true sense these substances are not water soluble but they swell up with the absorption of water.

Factors Governing Selection of an Ideal Ointment Base

A number of ointment bases have already been discussed but there is no ideal ointment base which fulfils all the requirements, since different types of bases are required for different purposes. A base suitable for normal skin may not be suitable for broken skin. Similarly a base suitable for dry skin may not be suitable for greasy skin. The factors which may help in the selection of an ideal ointment base are discussed below :

1. Dermatological factors
2. Pharmaceutical factors.

1. Dermatological Factors

(a) Absorption and Penetration

The word 'absorption' means actual entry into the blood stream, i.e., systemic absorption whereas 'penetration' means transference through the skin, i.e., cutaneous penetration.

Various experiments have been conducted by a number of scientists to study the problems of absorption and penetration which may be summarised as follows :

(i) Only the ointment base penetrates deep into the tissues of the skin.

(ii) It is mainly medicament which is absorbed into the blood stream.

(iii) Paraffins do not readily penetrate the skin whereas animal and vegetable fats and oils normally penetrate the skin. Animal fats, e.g., lard and wool fat when combined with water, penetrates the skin.

(iv) Substances which are soluble both in oil and water are most readily absorbed.

(v) Water soluble substances are more readily absorbed from water soluble bases.

(vi) O/W emulsion bases release the medicament more readily than greasy bases or W/O emulsion bases.

(b) Effect on Skin Function

Greasy bases interfere with normal skin functions, i.e., heat radiation and sweat. They are irritant to the skin. O/W emulsion bases and other water miscible bases produce a cooling effect rather than heating effect and mix readily with skin secretions.

(c) Miscibility with Skin Secretions and Serum

Skin secretions are more readily miscible with emulsion bases than with greasy bases. Due to this miscibility the drug is more rapidly and completely released to the skin hence lesser proportion of the medicament is required when such bases are used.

O/W emulsion bases are more readily miscible with serum from broken skin therefore they are particularly useful in weeping eczema.

(d) Compatibility with Skin Secretions

The bases used should be compatible with skin secretions and should have a pH about 5.5 because the average pH of the skin secretions is around 5.5. Generally neutral ointment bases are preferred.

(e) Freedom from Irritant Effect

Ointment bases used should be free from irritant effect on the skin. All bases used should be of high standard of purity and bases used specially for eye ointments should be non-irritating and free from foreign particles.

(f) Emollient Properties

Dryness and brittleness of the skin causes discomfort to the skin therefore the bases used should possess emollient properties that they should be able to keep the skin moist. For this purpose water and humectants such as glycerin and propylene glycol are used. Ointments containing wool fat, lard and liquid paraffin also act as emollients by preventing rapid loss of moisture from the skin.

(g) Ease of Application and Removal

The ointment bases used should be easily applicable as well as easily removable from the skin. Stiff and sticky ointments are not suitable as they may cause damage to the newly formed tissues of the skin. Therefore emulsion bases are more preferred as they are softer and spread more readily over the area to which they are applied. They can be easily removed by simply washing with water.

2. Pharmaceutical Factors

(a) Stability

Fats and oils obtained from animal and vegetable sources are liable to undergo oxidation unless they are suitably preserved. Lard, an animal fat used to be a common ingredient of ointments but it is rarely used now a days because it easily gets rancid. Soft paraffin, simple ointment and paraffin ointment are inert and stable. Liquid paraffin is also stable but on prolonged storage it gets oxidised therefore an antioxidant like tocopherol may be incorporated. Emulsions prepared with wool fat are liable to surface discolouration. O/W type emulsion bases provide a good medium for growth of microorganisms, therefore must be suitably preserved.

(b) Solvent Properties

Most of the medicaments used in the preparation of ointments are insoluble in the ointment bases therefore they are finely powdered and distributed uniformly throughout the base. Phenol, if dispersed in finely powdered state may cause blisters therefore it must be dispersed in a suitable base which should keep the phenol in solution form. Hence a base consisting of a mixture of hard paraffin, soft paraffins, bees wax and lard is used for this purpose. Similarly in the case of compound mercury ointment, olive oil is used to keep the camphor in solution form.

(c) Emulsifying Properties

Hydrocarbon bases can absorb only a small amount of aqueous substances whereas some animal fats can absorb an appreciable amount of water, e.g., wool fat can take up about 50% of water, and when mixed with other fats can take up several times its own weight of aqueous or hydroalcoholic liquids. Hence wool fat is included in the base for eye ointments.

Emulsifying ointment, cetrimide emulsifying ointment and cetomacrogol emulsifying ointment are capable of absorbing considerable amount of water, forming oil in water creams.

(d) Consistency

The ointments produced should be of suitable consistency. They should neither be too hard nor too soft. They should withstand the climatic conditions. Thus in summer they should not become too soft and in winter not too hard to be difficult to remove from the container and spread on the skin.

The consistency of an ointment can be adjusted by incorporating a suitable proportion of high melting point substances like hard paraffin, bees wax, etc., in too soft ointment; and low melting point substances like liquid paraffin in too hard ointments respectively.

Preparation of Ointments

There are two methods of preparation of ointments for extemporaneous compounding :

1. Trituration method
2. Fusion method.

1. Trituration Method

It is the most commonly and widely used method for the extemporaneous preparation of ointments. The medicaments which are to be incorporated in the base are generally insoluble in it, therefore it becomes necessary to reduce the medicament to fine powder otherwise the distribution of the medicament into the base will not be uniform.

In order to obtain the best results the medicament(s) is triturated with a small amount of the base on an ointment slab with the help of a stainless steel spatula with long broad blade. To this the additional quantities of the base are incorporated and triturated until the medicament(s) is homogeneously mixed with the base. To remove the gritty particles the ointment should be passed through an ointment mill.

When large volumes of liquids are to be incorporated, pestle and mortar should be used for the purpose. Relatively large amount of liquids can be incorporated by adding them gradually to an absorption base and then adding the fatty base. The pestle and mortar method is not as efficient as the slab method because :

(a) Certain particles have a tendency to slip out from under the pestle and thus the effect is not so pronounced.

(b) The sides of pestle and mortar will have to be scrapped from time to time.

Rx

Calamine, finely sifted	15 gm
White soft paraffin	85 gm

Label : The calamine ointment prepared by trituration method.

Procedure

Pass the calamine through a very fine sieve to get a fine powder. Triturate the calamine with a portion of white soft paraffin on an ointment slab with ointment spatula, until smooth. Gradually add the remainder of white soft paraffin with continuous trituration until a uniform ointment is obtained.

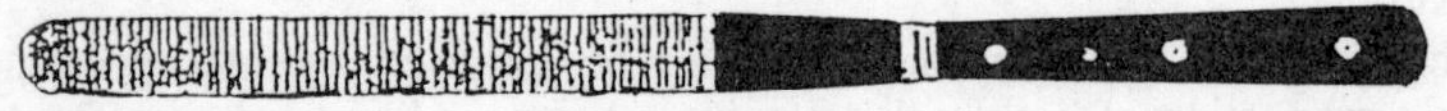

Fig. 9.1 Ointment spatula.

Pack the ointment in a wide mouth container or in an ointment jar, label and dispense. The container must be labelled with directions "For external use only.".

Uses

Calamine has a mild astringent action on the skin and is used in ointments to relieve discomfort of dermatitis.

2. Fusion Method

When an ointment base contains a number of solid ingredients such as white bees wax, cetyl alcohol, stearyl alcohol, stearic acid, hard paraffin, etc., as components of the base, it is necessary to melt them. The melting of the substances should be done in the decreasing order of their melting points, i.e., the substance with highest melting point should be melted first, then the substances with next melting point and so on. This will avoid the overheating of substances having low melting points. The medicament is then added slowly in the melted ingredients and stirred thoroughly until the mass cools down and a homogenous product is formed.

If any liquid or aqueous substance is also to be incorporated, that must be heated to about the same temperature as the melted bases. If it is not done so, then upon mixing the two portions the waxes or the solids will cool down quickly and they will solidify thereby they will prevent the homogeneous incorporation of the ingredients.

After melting the ingredients and mixing the two portions they should be stirred uniformly and thoroughly until homogeneous mass is obtained. Rapid cooling, i.e., by transferring into another cold container, cooling under tap water, using cold spatula or stirrer should be avoided because this will lead to the formation of solid lumps and a uniform product will not be obtained. When the ointment has begun to thicken, vigorous stirring should be avoided because this will lead to excessive entrainment of air in the ointment.

Sometimes due to the rapid cooling of the melted materials the waxy solids separate out and a uniform product is not obtained. To get a homogeneous product it can be remelted over a low heat and again stirred until cold.

Due to the greasy nature of many of the constituents of ointment bases they have the tendency to pick up dust and other foreign particles which are visible after melting the base. They can either be removed by decanting or passing through a piece of muslin which is kept in a warmed funnel or strainer and the clarified liquid is collected in another hot container.

Rx

Cetrimide	1 gm
Cetostearyl alcohol	10 gm
White soft paraffin	10 gm
Liquid paraffin	29 gm
Purified water	50 gm

Make an ointment.

Label : The antiseptic cream.

Type : Cream prepared by fusion method.

Procedure

Melt cetostearyl alcohol, white soft paraffin and liquid paraffin together. Separately dissolve cetrimide in purified water and warm it to almost same temperature (about 60°C) as that of melted substances. Add the warmed aqueous liquid to the melted mixture and stir thoroughly until cold. Pack in suitable container, label and dispense.

Uses

It is used as an antiseptic cream for the treatment of wounds and burns; for the pre-operative cleansing of the skin and for the removal of scabs and crusts in skin diseases.

Cetrimide is a quaternary ammonium compound. It is relatively non-toxic antiseptic with detergent properties. It is quite effective against gram-positive micro-organisms but less effective against gram-negative micro-organisms. Aqueous solutions containing 0.1 to 1.0% cetrimide are quite commonly used in hospitals.

3. Preparation of Ointments by Chemical Reaction

Some of the ointments like strong mercuric nitrate ointment and oleated mercury ointment were prepared by chemical reaction but now a days ointments containing free iodine or combined iodine are commonly prepared by this method.

(a) Ointments Containing Free Iodine

Iodine is slightly soluble in most fats and oils but is readily soluble in aqueous solutions of potassium iodide due to the formation of molecular compounds, e.g., $KI \cdot I_2$, $KI \cdot 2I_2$, $KI \cdot 3I_2$, according to the concentration of iodine present.

These complexes are not only soluble in water but they are also soluble in alcohol and glycerin. While dissolving it must be ensured that the liquid used should be non-volatile, otherwise the distributed medicament may crystallize when the solvent evaporates and these particles in the finished ointment will lead to irritation. Due to this reason sometimes glycerin is used as solvent instead of water which will not evaporate and prevent the formation of crystals.

The aqueous solutions so formed may be incorporated in absorption type bases to get an ointment. Strong iodine ointment B. Vet. C (British Vet. Codex) is prepared in this way. This ointment is used to treat ringworm infestation in cattle. Some time back such ointments were used in human beings but they badly stained the skin with deep red colour therefore were not popular. Due to this reason non-staining iodine is used now a days.

Exercise

Prepare 100 gm of strong iodine ointment B. Vet. C.

Formula :

Iodine
Wool fat
Yellow soft paraffin
Potassium iodide
Water

Procedure

Dissolve the potassium iodide in water. To this dissolve the iodine.

Separately melt wool fat and yellow soft paraffin together in a container, over water bath. Cool the melted mass to about 40°C. Add the iodine solution to the melted mass in small quantities at a time with continuous stirring until a uniform mass is obtained. Cool to room temperature and pack in glass jars. Plastic jars should not be used because iodine reacts with certain plastics.

Ointments Containing Combined Iodine

Fixed oils and many fats obtained from vegetable and animal sources can absorb iodine. This is due to the presence of unsaturated constituents in oils and fats which combine with iodine.

Paraffins which are generally used for the preparation of non-staining iodine ointment, under normal conditions, can absorb only 2% iodine because they consist almost entirely of saturated compounds while most fixed oils can combine with almost an equal weight of iodine, and some others can absorb much more than this amount. Under the conditions used for preparing these types of ointments, maximum absorption of iodine is not attained, therefore the quantity of oil used is much more than the theoretical quantity.

Although these ointments are dark, greenish-black in colour but leave no stain when rubbed into the skin as they are readily absorbed and leave no stain, therefore, they are known as non-staining iodine ointments.

Exercise

Prepare 100 gm of non-staining iodine ointment B.P.C. 1968.

Formula :

Iodine	50 gm
Arachis oil	150 ml
Yellow soft paraffin a sufficient quantity	

Procedure

Finely powder the iodine in a glass mortar and add the required amount in arachis oil contained in a glass-stoppered conical flask and stir well. Heat the flask at 50°C preferably in a thermostatically controlled water bath with occasional stirring until the brown colour changes to greenish-black.

Determine the concentration of iodine as stated in the B.P.C. and calculate the amount of soft paraffin required to produce a product of the required strength.

Warm the required amount of yellow soft paraffin to 40°C in a water bath. To this add the dissolved iodine with continuous stirring.

Pour the mixed mass into a warm container and allow to cool without stirring. Otherwise air will be entrapped and the product will become opaque.

4. Preparation of Ointments by Emulsification

An emulsion system must contain an emulsifying agent if they are to remain stable for sufficiently long time. Water soluble soaps were commonly used as emulsifiers for semisolid oil in water emulsions. The viscosity of ointments or creams prevents coalescence of the emulsified phases and helps to stabilize the emulsion. The addition of cetyl alcohol and glyceryl monostearate tends to stabilize the semi-solid oil in water emulsion whereas addition of polyvalent ions such as magnesium, calcium and aluminium tend to stabilize water in oil emulsions. Nearly all semi-solid creams and emulsified ointments require a combination of emulsifiers. Due to this reason a combination of triethanolamine stearate soap and cetyl alcohol is used as an emulsifier in oil in water emulsions and a combination of bees wax and divalent calcium ions is used as an emulsifier for water in oil emulsions.

The non-ionic emulsifiers like glyceryl monostearate, glyceryl mono-oleate, propylene glycol stearate, etc., are used for oil in water as well as water in oil emulsified semi-solids because they are compatible with most of the drugs. They can be used with strongly acidic salts or with strong electrolytes.

General Method of Preparation

In the preparation of ointments having an emulsion type formula, e.g., cold cream, the general method of preparation involves the melting process as well as an emulsification process.

In this method the water immiscible components such as oils, fats and waxes are melted together over water bath at a temperature of 70°C in an open vessel. Separately, the aqueous solution of all of the heat stable, water soluble components is heated to almost the same temperature as that of melted bases. Then this solution is slowly added to the melted bases, with continuous stirring until the product cools down and a semi-solid mass in obtained.

It is very important to heat the aqueous liquid to almost the same temperature as that of the melted bases otherwise high melting point fats and waxes will immediately solidify on addition of cold aqueous solution to the melted bases or vice versa, and a lumpy product will be obtained.

Other Additives in Ointments

In addition to the medicinal agent and the base other additives such as preservatives, antioxidants, chelating agents and perfumes may be incorporated in the ointment. Preservatives such as methyl paraben or propyl paraben may be incorporated to prevent the bacterial growth in the ointments which are to be stored for a long time. Antioxidants should be added whenever there are chances of oxidative decomposition of the ingredients. Similarly chelating agents can be included to prevent the catalytic oxidative degradation by trace elements. To retard the loss of moisture from the preparation, any humectant such as glycerin, propylene glycol or sorbitol may be added. Perfumes may also be incorporated to the ointments to give it a pleasant odour. A perfume blend which should be compatible with other components of the preparation should be added.

Other Related Dermatological Preparations

Creams

Creams are viscous semisolid ointment like preparations but have lighter body than the ointments. They may be oil in water type (aqueous creams) or water in oil type (oily creams). Due to the presence of water soluble bases in oil in water type creams they can be easily removed from the skin and clothings. The aqueous creams have a tendency to bacterial and mold growth, therefore a preservative must be added. Even if a preservative has been incorporated care must be taken for complete cleanliness of the apparatus used in the manufacture of creams and containers used for packing the creams. If this precaution is not observed and a cream contaminated with microorganisms is applied to the broken skin may produce infection in the patient.

Preparation of Creams

To prevent any contamination with micro-organisms the apparatus used in the preparation of creams must be thoroughly cleaned with soap and water and rinsed with freshly boiled and cooled water and finally dried in the oven. All hygienic precautions should be taken throughout the preparation and final transfer into the containers.

Containers and Storage

Creams should be supplied in well closed containers, which should prevent evaporation and contamination. They should be stored in a cool place. The collapsible tubes made of metals or plastics are most suitable for packing the creams. Ointment jars can also be used. Aluminium tubes are not suitable for packing creams which are preserved with an organic mercury compound.

Marketed Creams

1. Betnovate-N skin cream (Glaxo India Ltd., Bombay - 400025).

   Contains :

   Betamethasone valerate 0.12%
   Neomycin sulphate 0.5%

2. Caladryl cream [Parke-Davis (India) Ltd., Bombay - 400025].

   Contains :

   Calamine 8%

Camphor	0.1%
Diphenhydramine HCl	1%

3. Cetrimide cream (Alpine Industries, New Delhi - 110028).

Each contains :

Cetrimide	5 gm
Cetostearyl alcohol	50 gm
Purified water	445 gm
Liquid paraffin	500 gm

4. Dettol antiseptic cream (Reckitt & Colman of India Ltd., Calcutta - 700071).

Contains :

Chloroxylenol	0.8% W/W

5. Savlon antiseptic cream (ICI India Ltd., Madras - 600008).

Contains :

Cetrimide	0.5% W/W
Chlorhexidine HCl	0.1% W/W

6. Silver sulphadiazine cream (Duphar-Interfran Ltd., Bombay - 400018).

Each Contains :

Silver sulphadiazine	1% W/W

7. Sofradex cream (Roussel India Ltd., Bombay - 400018).

Contains :

Dexamethasone acetate	0.1% W/W
Framycetin sulphate	1.0% W/W

8. Soframycin skin cream (Roussel India Ltd., Bombay - 400018).

Contains :

Framycetin sulphate	1% W/W

Cerates

Cerates are semisolid ointment like preparations, containing a high percentage of wax which do not allow it to melt when applied to the skin. For its application they are usually spread on a material with cloth backing and then applied to the skin.

Plasters

Plasters are solid or semi-solid self-adhesive substances applied to the skin for protection, mechanical support or enhance the intimate contact between the drug and the skin. For its preparation the mass is melted and the drug is incorporated. Then the mixed mass is rolled into sticks and spread upon cloth, paper, linen or plastic. They are cut into different shapes according to the needs. The commonly used plasters are back plasters, breast plasters, chest plasters, corn plasters, and kidney plasters. Self-adhesive plaster (or tape) is the most extensively used preparation of this type. It does not require warming before application because it sticks closely to the skin at body temperature.

Marketed Adhesive Plasters

1. Adhesia adhesive plaster (Ranbaxy Labs Ltd., New Delhi - 110019).
2. Belladonna plaster (Johnson & Johnson).
3. Leucoplast (Beiersdorf India Ltd., Ponda, Goa).

Packing, Labelling and Storage of Ointments

Packing

The ointments are generally packed in ointment jars or collapsible tubes. Different shapes, types and capacities of ointment jars are used. They are made up of colourless or coloured glass. Amber coloured glass jars are used for light-sensitive preparations. While filling the ointment jars care must be taken to avoid the entrainment of air. The jars are so filled that the ointment is forced down along its sides so that no air is entrapped. Further the ointment jars are so filled to the surface that the cap or closure does not come in contact with the ointment.

Collapsible tubes made up of tin are also used for filling the ointments. For this purpose automatic machines are used. When so filled the ointments are less exposed to air, hence the chances of oxidation and contamination are reduced and preparations are likely to be more stable than the jar filled ointments. They are more hygienic because they are not contaminated by the fingers of the patient during its use. The collapsible tubes are also supplied with the applicators. So for easy application the cap can be removed from the container and applicator attached thereon.

Storage

The ointments should be stored in well closed containers and in a cool place. High temperatures are likely to soften or melt the bases during storage thereby rendering the preparation unfit for use.

Labelling

Ointment jars should be labelled with good quality of self-adhesive labels. As an additional precaution cello-tape can be wrapped around the label. Collapsible tubes should be labelled to the top because during use the tube is rolled up and this will prevent the spoilage of the label until the tube is practically empty. Self-adhesive strip labels are used because the ordinary gummed labels do not stick well to the surface of the container. Ointment tubes may be protected by placing them in cardboard boxes and the box labelled with additional label.

Stability of Ointments

The ointments should remain stable from the time of preparation to the time when whole of it is consumed.

On long storage the ointments lead to microbial growth therefore a suitable preservative must be added to inhibit the growth of contaminating micro-organisms. The preservatives must be selected very carefully. They should not react with the components of the formulations as well as the containers. Plastic containers may absorb the preservative and thereby decrease the quantity of preservative available for inhibiting or killing the micro-organisms responsible for spoilage of the preparation. The commonly used preservatives for ointments include p-hydroxybenzoates, phenol, benzoic acid, sorbic acid, methyl paraben, propyl paraben, quaternary ammonium compounds, mercury compounds, etc. The semisolid preparations which contain water in one way or the other are more prone to microbial growth. Therefore special care must be taken regarding their preservation.

Some ingredients like wool fat and its derivatives lead to oxidation. Therefore an antioxidant may be added to protect the active ingredients from oxidation.

Incompatibilities between drugs, emulsifying agents and preservatives must be avoided. The drugs which are likely to hydrolyse must be dispensed in an anhydrous base.

Humectants such as glycerin, propylene glycol and sorbitol may be added to prevent the loss of moisture from the preparation. Pigments such as iron oxides may be added to give ointments a cosmetic like appearance particularly for those preparations which are meant for application to the face.

Ointments must be stored at an optimum temperature otherwise separation of phases may take place in the emulsified products which may be very difficult to remix to get a uniform product.

Marketed Ointments

1. Burnol ointment (Boots Pharmaceuticals Ltd., Bombay - 400038).

   Contains :

   Aminovine HCl, Thymol.

2. Ledercort 0.1% skin ointment (Cyanamid India Ltd., Lederle Division, Bombay - 400025).

   Contains :

   Triamcinolone acetonide 0.1%

3. Ledercort-N skin ointment (Cyanamid India Ltd., Lederle Division, Bombay - 400025).

   Each contains :

   Triamcinolone acetonide 0.1%
   Neomycin sulphate 0.5% in vanishing cream.

4. Minit Medirub for colds (Geoffrey Manners & Co. Ltd., Bombay - 400038).

   Contains :

Camphor	6%
Menthol	3.1%
Thymol	1.0%
Methyl salicylate	1.0%
Turpentine oil	2.0%
Eucalyptus oil	2.0%

5. Myolaxin sports ointment (Geno Pharmaceuticals Ltd., Bombay - 400008).
6. New ring-cutter ointment (Jagsonpal Pharmaceuticals Ltd., New Delhi - 110016).

   Each gm contains :

Salicylic acid	10%
Benzoic acid	7.4%

7. Scabizan ointment (Zandu Pharmaceuticals Works Ltd., Bombay - 400025).

   Contains :

Precipitated sulphur	4%
Zinc oxide	4%
Salicylic acid	9%
Benzyl benzoate	15%

Pastes

Like ointments, pastes are the semisolid preparations meant for external application to the skin. They differ from ointments that they generally contain a large amount of finely powdered solids such as starch, zinc oxide, calcium carbonate, etc. Due to the presence of these substances they usually become quite thick and stiff than the ointments but are less greasy than ointments. Due to the presence of large amount of solids they are less attractive cosmetically than ointments.

Since pastes are stiff they do not melt at ordinary temperature thus forming and holding a protective coating over the areas to which they are applied. They soothen the inflamed and raw surfaces and in particular minimize the damage done by scratching in itching conditions such as chronic eczema. It is easier to stick the pastes to the diseased areas rather than ointments which are generally less viscous than pastes and tend to spread on to the healthy skin which may result in sensitivity reactions if the preparation contains a powerful medicament such as dithranol.

Pastes are prepared in the same manner as that of ointments but when a levigating agent is to be used to mix the components and to make the preparation smooth, a portion of the base should be used as levigating agent rather than a liquid like mineral oil that would soften the paste.

Pastes were originally formulated on the principle that the high contents of powder substances would absorb exudate but it is unlikely that a powder which has been specially wetted with oil will be able to absorb an aqueous liquid.

Pastes can be applied to the affected part with the help of a spatula or they may be spread on any of the dressing material and then applied. They are not removed from the site of application for quite a long time. The pastes are not suitable for application to the scalp because they are very difficult to remove from the hair.

Zinc and salicylic acid paste which is also known as Lessar's paste is the most commonly used paste. Medicaments incorporated in zinc and salicylic acid paste are less active than when included in ointments. Higher concentrations of powerful medicaments such as dithranol may therefore be tolerated if they are combined in zinc and salicylic acid paste.

Rx

Starch, finely sifted	24 gm
Zinc oxide, finely sifted	24 gm
Salicylic acid, finely sifted	2 gm
White soft paraffin	50 gm

Make a paste. Send 25 gm.

Label : The Lassar's paste.

Type : Paste with semisolid base prepared by fusion method.

Procedure

Melt the white soft paraffin on water bath. Incorporate the starch zinc oxide and salicylic acid which has been previously sifted through sieve no. 120. Stir until cold and homogeneous paste is obtained.

Rx

Dithranol	0.1	gm
Zinc and salicylic acid paste q.s.	100	gm

Make a paste. Send 25 gm.

Label : The dithranol paste.

Type : Paste prepared by trituration method.

Procedure

Warm the ointment slab because this preparation is best prepared on warm ointment slab. Triturate the weighed amount of dithranol with a small quantity of zinc and salicylic acid paste until smooth and complete dispersion is obtained. Gradually add the remainder of the zinc and salicylic acid paste with constant trituration until whole of it is added. Check the preparation to ensure that the dithranol is completely dispersed.

Bases Used for Pastes

The bases used for the preparation of pastes are as follows :

1. Hydrocarbon bases
2. Water miscible bases
3. Water soluble bases.

1. Hydrocarbon Bases

Soft paraffins and liquid paraffin are commonly used bases for the preparation of pastes. Compound zinc paste and compound zinc and salicylic acid paste are prepared with soft paraffin base. They are used in eczema and psoriasis either alone or along with coal tar and dithranol. Coal tar paste is used for treating eczema whereas dithranol paste is used for ringworm or psoriasis. Liquid paraffin is used as a base in compound aluminium paste which is used as skin protectant.

Rx

Zinc oxide, finely sifted	25 gm
Starch, finely sifted	25 gm
White, soft paraffin	50 gm

Make a paste. Send 25 gm.

Label : Spread thickly on white lint and apply to the affected area.

Type : Paste with semi-solid base prepared by fusion and trituration method.

Procedure

Separately pass the zinc oxide and starch through sieve no. 120. Melt the white soft paraffin on water bath. Mix the required weight of powders in a warm mortar. Add small amount of melted base with continuous trituration until smooth. Gradually add remainder of the base and mix until cold and uniform paste is obtained.

Uses

It is used as an antiseptic paste.

Note :

1. Warm mortar is used because it is much easier to manipulate the paste in warm mortar.
2. This preparation is also known as compound zinc paste.

Rx

Aluminium powder	20 gm

Zinc oxide	40 gm
Liquid paraffin	40 gm

Make a paste. Send 25 gm.
Label : The compound aluminium paste.
Type : Paste with liquid base prepared by trituration method.

Procedure

Mix aluminium powder and zinc oxide in a mortar. To this incorporate liquid paraffin and triturate thoroughly until smooth.

2. Water Miscible Bases

Emulsifying ointment is used as a base for resorcinol and sulphur paste. This paste is used in the treatment of dandruff therefore it should be easily removed from the hair, hence emulsifying ointment base is used.

Rx

Resorcinol, finely sifted	1.25 gm
Precipitated sulphur	1.25 gm
Zinc oxide, finely sifted	10.00 gm
Emulsifying ointment	12.50 gm

Fiat : Pasta. Mitte 50 gm.
Type : Paste containing semi-solid base and prepared by trituration method.

Procedure

Pass separately the resorcinol, precipitated sulphur and zinc oxide through sieve no. 120 and mix the weighed quantities of these substances with a portion of emulsifying ointment until smooth. Gradually add the remainder of the emulsifying ointment with thorough trituration until smooth.

Uses

It is used in the treatment of dandruff, psoriasis (chronic skin disease in which red scaly patches develop), eczema and other skin diseases.

Emulsifying wax is used in the preparation of zinc and coal tar paste which helps in easy dispersion of the coal tar as well as easy removal from the skin after use.

Magnesium sulphate paste is prepared by using glycerin as base to which phenol is added. This paste is used for the treatment of boils because of the powerful osmotic effects of magnesium sulphate and glycerin.

Titanium dioxide paste is prepared by using glycerin and water as base. This paste is a suspension which contains titanium dioxide, zinc oxide, light kaolin, red ferric oxide, glycerin and water. It is useful for absorbing exudates from weeping skin conditions.

3. Water Soluble Bases

Water soluble bases are prepared from mixtures of high and low molecular weight polyethylene glycols. The polyethylene glycols with low molecular weight are liquid in nature whereas the polyethylene glycols with a moderately higher molecular weight are semisolid and polyethylene glycols with higher molecular weight are solids. Suitable combinations of high and low molecular weight polyethylene glycols are mixed together to get a product of desired consistency which soften or melt when applied to the skin. These bases are water soluble because of the presence of many polar groups and ether linkages.

Water soluble dental paste containing neomycin sulphate is prepared with macrogol base. Another paste contains sodium carboxy methyl cellulose, pectin and gelatin is plastibase.

Methods of Preparation of Pastes

Like ointments, pastes are prepared by trituration and fusion methods. Trituration method is used when the base is liquid or semisolid while fusion method is used when the base is semisolid and/or solid in nature. These two methods have already been discussed in detail under methods of preparation of ointments.

Preservation of Pastes

Pastes which contain water as one of the ingredients (e.g., titanium dioxide paste) or fermentable ingredients, must be suitably preserved by adding anti-microbial preservatives. They should be stored in air-tight containers so as to prevent evaporation of moisture present in the paste.

Marketed Pastes

1. Zinc and salicylic acid paste (Lessar's paste) (Agrawal Pharmaceuticals, Delhi - 110092).
2. Zinc and salicylic acid paste (Lessar's paste) (Alpine Industries, New Delhi - 110028).
3. Magnesium sulphate ointment (Agrawal Pharmaceuticals, Delhi - 110092).

Jellies

Jellies are thin transparent or translucent non-greasy semisolid preparations meant for external application to the skin or mucous membrane. They are similar to mucilages because they may be prepared from gums similar to those used for mucilages but they differ from mucilages in having jelly like consistency. They are chiefly used on mucous membranes for their lubricating, antiseptic or spermicidal purposes. Jellies are also used for lubricating surgical gloves, catheters and rectal thermometers. Vaginal jellies and contraceptive jellies are also commonly used.

Medicated jellies contain a considerable amount of water therefore they are quite suitable as vehicles for water soluble medicaments such as local anaesthetics, spermicides and antiseptics. They are less satisfactory for insoluble medicaments which are difficult to incorporate and do not produce a uniform and smooth product.

Jellies are easy to apply and the evaporation of water content produces a cooling sensation to the skin. After evaporation the contents remaining behind stick well to the applied area and give a protection. When the treatment is over they can be easily removed by washing with water. The jellies used as lubricants for articles to be inserted into sterile regions of the body such as bladder, etc., must be sterile.

Preparation of Jellies

Pharmaceutical jellies are usually prepared by adding a thickening agent such as tragacanth or carboxymethyl cellulose to an aqueous solution in which drug has been dissolved. The mass is triturated in a mortar until a uniform product is obtained. Whenever a dark coloured drug is to be used then glass pestle and mortar must be used. For the preparation of jellies a whole gum is preferred rather than powdered gum because the former gives a clear preparation of uniform consistency. The following jelling agents are used for the preparation of jellies :

(i) Tragacanth

Tragacanth was frequently used for the preparation of lubricating, medicated and contraceptive jellies. The amount of gum required for the preparation of such jellies depends on the use of the jelly. For lubricating jelly 2 to 3% is sufficient but for dermatological vehicles about 5% gum is required. For the incorporation of ichthammol, resorcinol, salicylic acid and other medicaments a bassorin paste containing tragacanth 5% is used.

Tragacanth jellies are sometimes called bassorin pastes because the hydrophilic component of tragacanth which forms a gel in water is known as bassorin.

When tragacanth is added to water particularly, vice versa a lumpy product is obtained due to agglomeration of sticky, poorly wettable particles, which is difficult to disperse. Therefore a dispersing agent like alcohol and/or glycerin and/or a volatile oil is used to get a homogeneous preparation.

Tragacanth jellies are becoming less popular because of the following reasons :

(a) They vary in viscosity because the gum is obtained from natural sources.

(b) After evaporation the film left on the skin tends to flake.

(c) They lose viscosity quickly outside the pH range of 4.5 to 7, e.g., if benzoic acid is used as a preservative.

(d) They can't be stored for a long time.
(e) They are prone to microbial growth.

Rx

Ichthammol	1.0 gm
Tragacanth, in powder	2.5 gm
Alcohol 90%	5.0 ml
Glycerin	1.0 gm
Purified water q.s.	50.0 gm

Make a jelly.
Directions : To be spread in a thin layer over the affected part.

Procedure

To take into consideration the losses calculate for 60 gm instead of 50 gm. Take a 100 ml wide mouthed jar, put alcohol in it and add tragacanth; the reverse order may lead to lump formation. Shake well to mix. To this add water as quickly as possible and shake immediately.

Separately mix ichthammol, glycerin and 10 ml water. Add this solution to the mucilage and shake well. Adjust the final weight by adding more of water, if required, and shake well. Pack in a well closed container.

2. Sodium Alginate

Sodium alginate jellies are used as lubricants and dermatological vehicles. For lubricants 1.5 to 2% and for dermatological vehicles 5 to 10% sodium alginate is used. To increase the viscosity traces of soluble calcium salt may be added but high concentrations salt out the sodium alginate. 2 to 4% alcohol, glycerin or propylene glycol is used as dispersing agent. Sodium alginate has an advantage over tragacanth that it is available in several grades of standardised viscosity.

3. Pectin

Pectin is a very good gelling agent and is used in the preparation of many types of jellies including edible jellies. Glycerin is used as a dispersing agent and humectant in dermatological jellies. Pectin acts as a very good medium for the bacterial growth, therefore jellies prepared with pectin must be suitably preserved. Jellies must be packed in well closed containers to prevent the loss of moisture by evaporation.

4. Starch

Starch in combination with other substances like gelatin and glycerin was commonly used for the preparation of jellies. Still a product known as starch glycerin prepared by heating wheat starch with water and glycerin is used. Starch mucilages prepared with water alone lead to bacterial growth therefore a suitable preservative must be added. Glycerin in large amounts, i.e., 50% may be included which will act as preservative and humectant. Medicaments are incorporated in the cold jelly by trituration. Starch jellies should be freshly prepared and packed in well closed containers to prevent the loss of moisture by evaporation.

5. Gelatin

Gelatin is insoluble in cold water but swells and softens in it. It is soluble in hot water. A hot solution containing only 2% gelatin forms a jelly on cooling. Very stiff medicated jellies can be prepared by incorporating about 15% gelatin. Such jellies are melted before use and after cooling to desired temperature are applied with a brush to the affected area. The area is covered with bandage and the dressing may be left in place for several weeks. Zinc gelatin jelly which is also known as Unna's paste is the main preparation of this type.

Rx

Prepare 100 gm zinc gelatin jelly.

Formula :

Zinc oxide	15 gm
Gelatin	15 gm
Glycerin	35 gm
Water	35 gm

Make a jelly. Send 50 gm.
Directions : Apply to the affected part as directed.

Procedure

Soak the gelatin in water until thoroughly softened, add the glycerin and heat over water bath until the gelatin is dissolved, adjust the weight to 850 gm, if necessary, by adding more of water.

Pass the zinc oxide through sieve no. 120 and weigh the required amount and add it in small amounts to the melted base with gentle stirring to avoid excessive incorporation of air. Continue stirring until a uniform viscous product is obtained.

Pour the product so obtained in a tray to a depth of about 1 cm, with continuous trituration throughout the operation. When the mass has set, carefully cut the mass into pieces of about 1.5 cm square, with a blade or sharp knife. Pack in well closed wide mouthed container.

If the jelly is poured directly into the container, sedimentation of zinc oxide may take place if the preparation is not stirred well each time when it is used. This may result in very uneven medication if the same jar containing the jelly is used for many patients or on several occasions. Dividing the product into small pieces is a convenient method where a desired number of pieces can be melted for each treatment, which will give a uniform composition.

6. Cellulose Derivatives

Methyl cellulose and sodium carboxy methyl cellulose are widely used for the preparation of jellies. These substances produce neutral jellies of very stable viscosity and afford good resistance against bacterial growth. These jellies are quite clear due to freedom from insoluble impurities and produce a strong film after drying on the skin. Sodium carboxy methyl cellulose is used for the preparation of lubricating jellies as well as used for sterile jellies such as lignocaine gel because it can withstand autoclaving without serious deterioration.

Preservation of Jellies

Although some bases used for the preparation of jellies, e.g., clays and cellulose derivatives, resist the bacterial attack but since all the jellies contain large amount of water therefore they must be suitably preserved by adding an antimicrobial preservative, unless they are to be used immediately. Methyl p-hydroxybenzoate 0.1 to 0.2% W/V is commonly used preservative for medicated jellies.

There is quick loss of water which leads to skin formation on jellies. Therefore to prevent this a hygroscopic substance such as glycerin, propylene glycol or sorbitol may be added.

Containers

Containers containing jellies should be well filled to minimise evaporation of water, well closed and stored in a cool place to prevent drying out.

Collapsible tubes should be used for packing the sterile products such as catheter lubricants.

Marketed Gels/Jellies

1. Candid-V gel (Glenmark Pharmaceuticals Ltd., Bombay - 400026).

   Each contains :

Clotrimazole	2%

2. Daktacort gel (NR Jet Enterprises Ltd., Bombay - 400078).

   Each contains :

Miconazole nitrate I.P.	2% W/W
Hydrocortisone acetate	1% W/W

3. Gyno-Daktarin gel (NR Jet Enterprises, Bombay - 400078).

   Each contains :

   Miconazole nitrate gel

4. Gentian violet jelly (Arora Pharmaceuticals Pvt. Ltd., New Delhi - 110035).
5. Thrombophob gel (German Remedies Ltd., Bombay - 400018).

   Each gm contains :

   Heparin Sod. 200 I.U.

Poultices

Poultices are also known as cataplasms. They are soft, viscous wet masses of solid substances applied to the skin for their fomentation action in order to give relief from pain or reduce inflammation or in some cases to act as counter-irritant. They are also used to draw infectious material from diseased tissues because of the absorptive and hygroscopic characters of the ingredients. They represent one of the most ancient classes of pharmaceutical preparations. Now a days the practising pharmacists never prepare poultices but sometimes may be asked to prepare such preparations. Clay metals such as heavy kaolin, herbs and seeds such as mustard, linseed, etc., are used for their preparation. Glycerin is incorporated because of its hygroscopic nature.

For use the poultice is heated in a dish with occasional stirring until the heat is tolerated on the back of the hand. Then it is spread thickly on a dressing material and applied as hot as the patient can bear it to the affected area which is sometimes first covered with muslin to facilitate removal after use. Only kaolin poultice is included in B.P. 1980.

Exercise

Prepare kaolin poultice 100 gm

Formula :

Heavy kaolin, finely sifted and dried at 100°C	52.7	gm
Boric acid, finely sifted	4.5	gm
Methyl salicylate	0.2	ml
Thymol	50	mg
Peppermint oil	0.05	ml
Glycerin	42.5	gm

Procedure

Mix heavy kaolin and boric acid with glycerin and heat at 120°C for one hour with occasional stirring, and allow to cool. Separately dissolve thymol in methyl salicylate and peppermint oil, add this solution to the cooled mixture and mix thoroughly.

Heavy kaolin is liable to be contaminated with bacterial spores like clostridium tetanii. Therefore it is necessary to heat kaolin at 120°C to kill these spores.

It cannot be heated beyond 120°C to prevent decomposition of glycerin.

Kaolin poultice is stored in well closed containers to prevent loss of volatile ingredients and absorption of moisture from the atmosphere by glycerin.

Marketed Poultice

1. Antigestine poultice (Agrawal Pharmaceuticals, Delhi - 110092).
2. Antiflamistin poultice (Arora Pharmaceuticals Pvt. Ltd., Delhi - 110035).
3. Ketolin antiplast poultice [Mehta Unani Pharmacy & Co., Rajkot - 360001, Gujarat].

Revision Questions

I. Very short answer type questions

(A) Define the following :

(a) Ointments
(b) Creams
(c) Pastes
(d) Jellies
(e) Ointment bases
(f) Cerates
(g) Plasters
(h) Poultices

(B) Fill in the blanks :

(a) Ointments are ...... preparations meant for ...... application to the skin.
(b) There are two methods of preparation of ointments namely ...... and ....
(c) Trituration method of preparation of ointments is used when the base is ...... and the medicament is ...... in the base.
(d) Fusion method of preparation of ointments is used when ointment base contains a number of ...... of different ....
(e) Hydrous wool fat or lanolin is a mixture of ...... wool ft and ...... purified water.

II. Short answer type questions

1. Write short notes on the following :

(a) Ointments
(b) Creams
(c) Pastes
(d) Jellies
(e) Ointment bases
(f) Cerates

(g) Plasters
(h) Poultices

2. Discuss the characteristics of an ideal ointment.
3. Give a brief account of oleaginous bases used in the preparation of ointments, also mention their disadvantages.
4. Name the absorption bases. Give the advantages and disadvantage of absorption bases.
5. Write in brief about methods of preparation of ointments.
6. Give in brief the packing, labeling and storage of ointments.
7. Differentiate between :
   (a) Ointments and creams
   (b) Ointments and pastes
   (c) Paste and jellies.
   (d) Poultice and jellies.
8. Discuss preservation and containers for jellies.
9. Name at least three marketed preparations of the following :
   (a) Ointments
   (b) Creams
   (c) Jellies

III. Long answer type questions

1. What are ointments? Explain how do they differ from pastes, creams and jellies.
2. Define an ointment base. Discuss the qualities of an ideal ointment base and describe various factors governing the selection of an ideal ointment base.
3. What is an ointment base? Classify and explain different types of ointment bases used. Discuss advantages and disadvantages of one base over the other.
4. Discuss various methods of preparation of ointments.
5. What are jellies? Discuss various types of jellies and describe in brief the formulation of jellies.
6. Give the method of preparation of the following :
   (a) Non-staining iodine ointment B.P.C. 1968.
   (b) Cetrimide cream
   (c) Zinc and salicylic acid paste i.e. 'lesser paste'.
   (d) Compound zinc paste.
   (e) Whitfield's ointment
   (f) Kaolin poultice
7. Explain the reasons for the following :
   (a) Why ointments and other preparations meant for external use should be free from gritty particles?

(b) Why heavy kaolin is heated at 120°C before its use in the preparation of kaolin poultice?
(c) Why non-staining iodine ointment leaves no stain on the skin when rubbed on the skin?
(d) Why white soft paraffin should not be used in the preparation of ophthalmic ointments?
(e) Why the liquid or aqueous substance to be incorporated in the melted oily bases are to be heated to almost same temperature as that of melted bases?

Answers

I. (B)
(a) Semisolid, external
(b) Trituration method, fusion method
(c) Soft or semisolid, insoluble
(d) Solid ingredients, melting points
(e) 70% W/W, 30% W/W

10

Suppositories

Suppositories are special shaped solid dosage form of medicament meant for insertion into body cavities other than mouth. They may be inserted into rectum, vagina or the urethra. These products are so formulated that after insertion, they will either melt or dissolve in the cavity fluids to release the medicament. Suppositories vary in shapes, sizes and weights. Generally suppositories weighing 1 to 2 gm are prepared. Cocoa butter or glycerogelatin is used as base.

Uses

Suppositories are used for any one of the three different purposes.

1. To produce local action.
2. To produce systemic action.
3. To produce mechanical action on the lower bowel and facilitate evacuation in the treatment of haemorrhoids, anal irritation, constipation, etc.

Suppositories are convenient mode of administration of drugs which irritate the gastro-intestinal tract, cause vomitting, are destroyed by the hepatic circulation, or are destroyed in the stomach by pH changes, enzymes, etc.

They can be easily administered to children, old persons and to unconscious patients who cannot swallow the drugs easily.

The rectal suppositories may be used for lubricating, soothing, antiseptic, local anaesthetic action or for astringent effect. Therefore they may contain antiseptics, local anaesthetics, astringents, hormones and steroids. The rectal suppositories meant for systemic effect contain analgesics, antispasmodics, sedatives and tranquilizers.

The lower portion of the rectum affords a large absorption surface area from which the soluble substances can pass quickly and reach the venous circulation directly and rapid action of the drug is produced. However the rate and extent of absorption of the drugs depends upon the nature of the base in which they have been incorporated. The maximum therapeutic effect is produced if the drug incorporated is in the finely divided state, evenly distributed throughout the base and in a readily absorbable form.

The rectal suppositories are extensively used as a mechanical aid to bowel evacuation which produce its action by irritating the mucous membrane of the rectum or by lubricating action. The glycerin suppositories are representative example of evacuant suppositories.

Types of Suppositories

1. Rectal Suppositories

These are meant for introduction into the rectum for their systemic effect. They are tapered at one or both ends and usually weigh about 2 gm. The rectal suppositories meant for children are smaller in size and weight than the adult suppositories. They usually weigh about 1 gm.

2. Vaginal Suppositories

They are also known as pessaries and are meant for introduction into the vagina. They are larger than rectal suppositories and vary in weight from 3 to 6 gm or more. The vaginal suppositories may be conical, rod-shaped or wedge-shaped. They are exclusively used for their local action on the vagina.

Special shaped suppositories are manufactured and are supplied with applicators to facilitate insertion into the vagina. Now a days a few special tablets and capsules, oval or suppository shaped are prepared for use in the vagina and are known as vaginal tablets and vaginal capsules respectively.

3. Urethral Suppositories

They are also known as urethral bougies and are meant for introduction into the urethra. They are long, thin and cylindrical forms rounded on one end. Their weight varies from 2 to 4 gm and length from 2 to 5 inch. Urethral suppositories are very rarely used.

4. Nasal Suppositories

They are also known as nasal bougies or buginaria and are meant for introduction into the nasal cavity. They are similar in shape to urethral bougies. Their weight is about 1 gm and length 9-10 cm. They are always prepared with glycero-gelatin base.

5. Ear Cones

They are also known as aurinaria and are meant for introduction into the ear. They are very rarely used. Generally theobroma oil is used as a base, prepared in an urethral bougies mould and cut according to the required size.

Newer Concept of Suppositories

Recently some newer concepts of suppositories regarding their formulation and packaging have been introduced which are described below :

1. Tablet Suppositories

Suppositories such as rectal suppositories and pessaries are formulated and prepared by compression like tablets. They contain disintegrating agents like effervescent combinations or starch. Pessaries are generally prepared as almond shape for ease in insertion and to provide a large surface area for disintegration and absorption. Rectal tablets are generally covered with thin layers of materials such as polyethylene glycol for protection and to facilitate insertion into the rectum.

2. Layered Suppositories

These types of suppositories contain different drugs in different layers. Thus the incompatible drugs can be separated from each other. Similarly drugs having different melting points or dissolution characteristics can be incorporated to control the absorption rates. These types of suppositories can be prepared by partially filling the mould with one type of material, when it congeals then the other materials are added as a separate layer and allowed to cool.

3. Coated Suppositories

Suppositories are given coatings with materials such as polyethylene glycols, cetyl alcohol, etc., to control their disintegration rate, to impart lubricant properties or to provide protective action during storage. For coating the suppositories are dipped in solutions of coating materials until coats of desired thickness have been obtained and then dried.

4. Capsule Suppositories

Soft gelatin capsules of different shapes and sizes are prepared for insertion into the rectum or the vagina. These types of capsules are increasing in popularity. Liquids, semisolids or solids can be filled in such capsules.

5. Packing in Disposable Moulds

Previously the suppositories prepared in metallic moulds or by compression method were individually wrapped and supplied in boxes. But in recent method the suppositories are directly made in disposable moulds made up of plastic materials or tin foils. The suppository mass is poured into the disposable moulds and cooled, the excess is trimmed off and the moulds are sealed, then they are packed in cartons. These types of moulds have the advantage that if due to any reason the mass melts it will remain in the mould itself which can be used after cooling.

Suppository Bases

Since suppositories are special solid dosage form of medicament they must retain its shape, solidity and firmness during storage and administration but melt or dissolve in the cavity fluids when inserted into the body cavity. Therefore the materials used as suppository bases must impart these properties and also fulfil other formulation requirements. There are a large number of bases used but theobroma oil, glycerogelatin base and polyethylene glycols fulfil the above mentioned requirements. An ideal suppository base should have the following properties :

1. It should be good in appearance.
2. It should melt at body temperature, dissolve or disperse in the body cavity fluids.
3. It should retain its shape when being handled.
4. It should be stable on storage, i.e., it should not undergo any physical or chemical change on storage.
5. It should be completely nontoxic and non-irritant to the mucous membrane of the body cavity.
6. It should release the incorporated medicament(s) readily.
7. It should be compatible with large number of drugs.
8. It should easily attain the shape of the mould and should not stick to the sides of the mould.
9. It should be easily mouldable by cold compression or by pouring in the cavities of the mould.
10. It should not decompose even if heated above its melting point.

Since it is not possible to get all the above mentioned qualities in a single base, so a combination of bases is used to get a product of required qualities. A number of patent "improved" suppository bases are available. Most of these are mixtures of fats, waxes and/or esters in specific proportions according to the desired qualities of the product to be obtained. Glycerogelatin and polyethylene glycols are being widely used as suppository bases, though theobroma oil is extensively used in extemporaneous preparations but it is losing its importance because it is unstable to heat and has undesirable physical properties.

Types of Suppository Bases

In general there are three types of suppository bases.

1. Oily bases
2. Water soluble and water miscible bases
3. Emulsifying bases.

Oily Bases

(i) Theobroma Oil

Theobroma oil is also known as cocoa butter. It is obtained from the crushed and roasted seeds of Theobroma Cocoa. It is a yellowish white solid which becomes white on storage. It has butter like consistency and chocolate like odour. It has a melting point of 30 to 35°C. It is a mixture of glyceryl esters of stearic, palmitic, oleic and other fatty acids.

Theobroma oil is most widely used suppository base since it melts at body temperature and release the medicament into the cavity fluids for rapid absorption. While theobroma oil is generally a very good base for rectal suppositories, it is not quite suitable for pessaries, urethral bougies or nasal bougies because after melting it has a tendency to leak out of the cavities and of its immiscibility with mucous secretions.

Cocoa butter has most of the qualities which an ideal suppository base should have but its main disadvantages are that (a) overheating changes its physical characteristics; (b) it has tendency to adhere to the sides of the mould when solidified. Polymorphism takes place when melted theobroma oil is solidified. Different crystalline forms formed depend upon the temperature of melting and rate of cooling. However a stable form is obtained if the melted mass is s allowed to cool slowly and stand for a few days in a cool place. The other disadvantages of cocoa butter are that it becomes rancid, melts in warm weather, liquefaction takes place when incorporated with certain drugs, immiscible with body fluids, failure to release the medicament and leakage from the body cavities.

(ii) Emulsified Theobroma Oil

Emulsified theobroma oil may be used as a base when large quantities of aqueous solutions are to be incorporated. Several agents have been used to form emulsified theobroma oil suppositories. The use of 5% glyceryl monostearate, 10% lanette wax, 2-3% cetyl alcohol, 4% bees wax and spermaceti up to 12% is recommended for emulsified theobroma oil suppositories.

(iii) Hydrogenated Oils

As a substitute of theobroma oil a number of hydrogenated oils, e.g., hydrogenated edible oil, coconut oil, palm kernel oil, hydrogenated pea oil, stearin and a mixture of oleic and stearic acids are recommended. Synthetic fat bases have a number of advantages over theobroma oil that :

(a) Overheating does not affect the solidifying point.
(b) They are resistant to oxidation.
(c) Their emulsifying and water absorbing capacities are good.
(d) Lubrication of the mould is not required.
(e) They produce colourless, odourless and elegant suppositories.

Synthetic fat bases also have disadvantages that (a) on rapid cooling in the refrigerator they become brittle; (b) when melted they are more fluid than theobroma oil and result in greater sedimentation of the added substances. This difficulty may be overcome by the addition of some thickening agent such as bentonite, magnesium stearate and colloidal silicon dioxide, etc.

2. Water Soluble and Water Miscible Bases

(a) Glycero-Gelatin

Glycero-gelatin base is a mixture of glycerin and water which is made stiff by the addition of gelatin. The stiffness of the mass depends upon the proportion of gelatin used which is adjusted according to the purpose for which the preparation is intended. This base has many properties that desirable suppositories can be prepared with it. The base being hydrophilic in nature, slowly dissolves in the aqueous secretions and provide a slow continuous release of medicament. This base may be used to prepare all types of suppositories but it is particularly used as vehicle in vaginal suppositories. Glycerogelatin base is well suited for suppositories containing belladonna extract, boric acid, chloral hydrate, bromides, iodides, iodoform, opium, etc.

Depending upon the compatibility of the drugs used a suitable type of gelatin is selected for the purpose. Two types of gelatins are used as suppository base (i) Type-A or pharmagel A which is acidic in nature is used for acidic drugs; and (ii) Type-B or pharmagel B which is alkaline in nature is used for alkaline drugs.

Disadvantages

Glycerogelatin base suppositories are less commonly used than the fatty base suppositories because :

(i) They are more difficult to prepare and handle.

(ii) They are hygroscopic therefore they must be stored in well closed containers.

(iii) Gelatin is incompatible with many drugs, e.g., tannic acid, ferric chloride, gallic acid, etc.

(iv) They support bacterial and mold growth therefore a preservative such as methylparaben and propylparaben must be added.

(v) The solution time depends on the content and quality of the gelatin used.

(b) Soap Glycerin Suppositories

In glycerogelatin base the gelatin is replaced with either curd soap or sodium stearate which makes the glycerin sufficiently hard for suppositories and a large quantity of glycerin up to 95% of the mass can be incorporated further the soap helps in the evacuation action of glycerin whereas gelatin does not.

The soap glycerin suppositories have disadvantage that they are very hygroscopic therefore they must be protected from atmosphere and wrapped in waxed paper or tin foil.

(c) Polyethylene Glycols

Polyethylene glycol polymers are widely used in the extemporaneous preparations and commercial manufacture of suppositories. They are commonly known as 'Carbowaxes' and 'Polyglycols'. Depending upon the molecular weight they are available in different physical forms. Polyethylene glycol polymers having the molecular weight between 200 to 1000 are liquids and those with molecular weight higher than 1000 are wax like solids. They are chemically stable and physiologically inert substances and do not allow the bacterial or mold growth to take place. Suppositories of varying melting points and solubilities can be prepared by using a blend of polyethylene glycols of different molecular weights.

3. Emulsifying Bases

These are synthetic bases and a number of proprietary bases of very good quality are available, a few of which are described below :

(a) Massa Esterinum

This is also known as adeps solidus. It is a mixture of mono, di and triglycerides of saturated fatty acids having the formula $C_{11}H_{23}COOH$ to $C_{17}H_{35}COOH$. It is a white, brittle, almost odourless and tasteless solid. It melts at 33.5 to 35.5°C. Several grades of massa esterinum are available but grade B is recommended for general dispensing.

(b) Witepsol

They consist of triglycerides of saturated vegetable acid with varying proportions of partial esters. A small amount of beeswax is added for use in hot climates.

Suppositories prepared with witepsol bases (i) should not be ice-cooled since they may become brittle and fracture if cooled too rapidly (ii) the mould must not be lubricated.

(c) Massuppol

It consists of glyceryl esters mainly of lauric acid, to which a small amount of glyceryl monostearate has been added to improve its water absorbing capacity.

The above mentioned synthetic compounds have advantages over cocoa butter that :

1. Overheating does not alter the physical characteristics.
2. They do not stick to the mould.
3. They do not require previous lubrication of the mould rather lubrication is a disadvantage as it may spoil the appearance of the suppositories.
4. They solidify rapidly.
5. They are less liable to get rancid.
6. They can absorb fairly large amount of aqueous liquids.

Preparation of Suppositories

Suppositories are prepared by three processes : rolling, moulding (hot process or fusion method) and cold compression. The hand rolling and shaping method is of historical importance and not used now a days.

Hot Process or Fusion Method

Mould

Various types and sizes of suppository moulds are available for commercial use. In the dispensary suppository moulds with six or twelve cavities with desired shape and size may be used. For large scale production moulds up to 500 cavities may be used. They are made up of stainless steel, nickel-copper alloy, brass, aluminium or plastic.

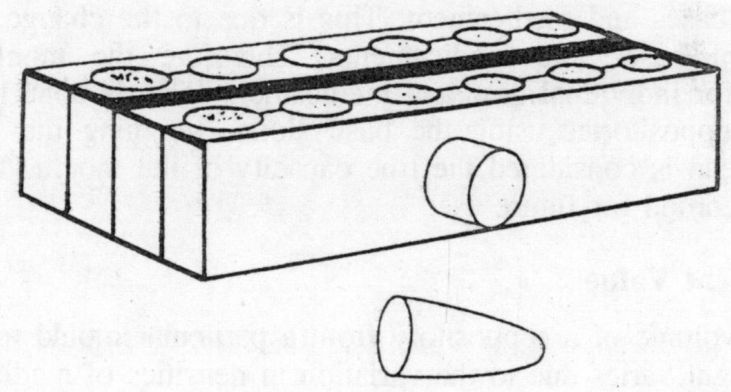

Fig. 10.1 Suppositories mould.

For cleaning, lubrication and removal of suppositories the mould can be opened longitudinally by removing the screw in the centre of the plates. For cleaning, the opened plates are immersed in hot water containing detergent, then they are washed with water and dried thoroughly. Care must be taken that the inner surface of the cavities do not have any scratch otherwise suppositories with uneven surface will be produced.

Lubrication of Moulds

Whenever cocoa butter or glycero-gelatin in used as a base for the preparation of suppositories it is necessary to lubricate the mould otherwise suppositories with smooth surface will not be obtained because of the sticky nature of these bases which will stick to the sides of the mould. The lubricant applied must be of different nature than the base, otherwise it will be absorbed and fail to provide a buffer film between the suppository and the metal of the mould. Therefore an oily lubricant for cocoa butter suppositories and aqueous lubricant for glycerogelatin suppositories is useless. So a lubricant containing soft soap 10 gm, glycerol 10 gm and alcohol (90%) 50 ml is most suitable for oily bases and liquid paraffin or arachis oil for glycero-gelatin suppositories respectively.

Whenever emulsifying bases or macrogol bases are used there is no need to lubricate the moulds. Products with better surface are obtained if the mould is kept dry.

For lubricating the moulds, the lubricant should be applied with the help of a brush or a swab made of gauze. Cotton wool should not be used because it detaches the fibres too easily. Excessive lubrication of the mould should be avoided, if it happens so, the mould should be closed and inverted on a white tile to drain the excessive lubricant out.

Calibration of the Mould

Unless otherwise stated a standard mould of 15 grain or 1 gramme capacity is used, but it is not wise to assume that the capacity of the mould is correct. Though the size remains same but the weight varies with the change of bases and medicament. This is due to the change in densities of different bases and medicaments. Therefore the mould must be calibrated for individual base and medicament. This is done by preparing a set of suppositories using the base alone, weighing the product and average mean is considered the true capacity of the mould. These values may be recorded for future use.

Displacement Value

Since the volume of a suppository from a particular mould remains same but its weight varies due to the variation in densities of medicaments and the base with which the mould was calibrated. To get a product of uniform and accurate weight, allowance must be made for the change in density of the mass due to added drugs. For this purpose the displacement value of the medicament is taken into consideration.

"The quantity of the drug which displaces one part of the base is known as displacement value."

Displacement values of some medicaments used in suppositories with reference to cocoa butter are given below :

Medicament	*Displacement value*
Aminophylline	1.5
Boric acid	1.5
Castor oil	1.0
Chloral hydrate	1.5
Cocaine hydrochloride	1.5
Hamamelis dry extract	1.5
Hydrocortisone acetate	1.5
Ichthammol	1.0
Iodoform	4.0
Morphine hydrochloride	1.5
Phenobarbitone	1.0
Tannic acid	1.0
Zinc oxide	5.0
Liquid medicaments	1.0

The use of displacement value in calculations is described in the following example :

Prepare 10 suppositories each containing 3 grains of iodoform. The displacement value of iodoform is 4.0.

Since the 15 grain weight suppository mould is used so the total weight of theobroma oil (alone) required for 10 suppositories

$= 15 \times 10 = 150$ gr.

The total quantity of iodoform required for 10 suppositories

$= 10 \times 3 = 30$ gr.

4 grain of iodoform displaces 1 gr. of theobroma oil.

1 grain of iodoform displaces ¼ gr. of theobroma oil.

∴ 30 grain of iodoform will displace $\frac{1}{4} \times 30$ gr. of theobroma oil

$= 7.5$ gr.

Therefore the actual quantity of cocoa butter required for preparing 10 suppositories will be $150 - 7.5 = 142.5$ gr.

The total weight of 10 suppositories will be $142.5 + 30 = 172.5$ gr., i.e., @ 17.25 gr. for each suppository.

It indicates that although the suppositories are made in 15 grain mould their volume remains same but the weight is much more than 15 grains. Therefore it is necessary to take into consideration the displacement value of the drug while calculating the quantity of the base for suppositories.

Determination of Displacement Value of Medicaments

The displacement value of a given medicament may be determined as follows :

(a) Prepare and weigh 10 suppositories containing theobroma oil alone (or other base). Let it be *a* gm.
(b) Prepare and weigh 10 suppositories containing 40% of medicament. Let it be *b* gm.
(c) Calculate the amount of theobroma oil present in the medicated suppositories. Let it be *c* gm.
(d) Calculate the amount of medicament present in the medicated suppositories. Let it be *d* gm.
(e) Calculate the amount of theobroma oil displaced by *d* gm of medicament. Let it be $(a - c)$ gm.

$$\text{Displacement value of medicament} = \frac{d}{(a-c)}$$

Example

Determine the displacement value of a medicament in theobroma oil suppositories containing 40% medicament, prepared in 1 gm mould. The weight of 10 suppositories is 14.66 gm.

Solution

(a) Weight of 10 suppositories containing theobroma oil alone prepared in 1 gm capacity mould = 1 × 10 = 10 gm.
(b) Weight of 10 suppositories containing 40% of medicament = 14.66 gm.
(c) Amount of theobroma oil present $= \frac{60}{100} \times 14.66 = 8.796$ gm.
(d) Amount of medicament present $= \frac{40}{100} \times 14.66 = 5.864$ gm.
(e) Amount of theobroma oil displaced by 5.864 gm of medicament = 10.0 – 8.796 = 1.204 gm.

∴ Displacement value of medicament $= \frac{5.864}{1.204} = 5$ (Approx.).

General Method of Preparation

Thoroughly clean and lubricate the mould with a suitable lubricant, keep it on ice in the inverted position to cool and drain any excess of the lubricant. The lubrication of the mould is unnecessary with synthetic bases.

Taking into account the displacement value of the medicament place the calculated quantities of powdered or shredded cocoa butter in a dish. (An excess must be calculated because of unavoidable wastage during preparation. For this the amount for two extra suppositories is sufficient, that means if eight suppositories are to be dispensed then calculate for ten suppositories instead of eight.) Heat the dish over water bath and when two-third of the base melts remove the dish from the bath and stir thoroughly until whole of the mass melts. This process prevents overheating of the base.

Place the weighed quantity of powdered medicament to be incorporated on a warmed ointment slab, over it put about half the melted base, rub it thoroughly with a flexible spatula, care must be taken to prevent the formation of lumps. Transfer the mixed mass to the dish and mix thoroughly so that a uniform mass is formed.

Warm the dish over water bath for few seconds with constant stirring until the mass becomes pourable. Transfer this melted mass rapidly into the cavities of the mould kept over ice. Fill each cavity to overflowing, this is done to prevent the formation of hollows in the tops of the finished suppositories because cocoa butter contracts on cooling and hollows are formed at the top of the suppositories. While pouring the mass into the cavities it must be continuously stirred to ensure even distribution of the medicament in all the suppositories.

When the mass has just set, remove the excess of the mass with the help of a sharp knife or razor blade or a slightly warmed spatula. Keep the mould in cool place or over ice for 10 to 15 minutes. Then open the mould and remove the suppositories. If any lubricant is there, wipe it off lightly with a clean cloth.

Cold Compression Method

This method has the advantage that it avoids heat and stirring therefore it is suitable for thermolabile and insoluble drugs. It is not suitable for suppositories in which glycerogelatin is used as base and other bases in which melting is necessary. In this method the mass is prepared by first mixing the powdered drug with an equal amount of grated cocoa butter and then incorporating the remaining amount of grated cocoa butter. Allowance is made for unavoidable wastage during preparation by calculating for sufficient extra suppositories.

The prepared mass C is placed in a cylinder A of the machine which is forced to the cavities of the mould through the narrow opening D by applying pressure to the piston B or handle of the machine thus forming suppositories at E. The pressure is further applied, stop plate F is removed and the finished suppositories are taken out. The working of the machine is shown in the diagram.

The operation is repeated for the next set of suppositories. On large scale manufacturing the hydraulically operated cold-compression machines are used which are cooled by water jackets to prevent the heat of compression from making the mass too fluid.

Packing and Storage

Suppositories are usually packed in shallow, partitioned cardboard boxes which hold the suppositories in upright position and do not allow them to come in contact with each other. If plain boxes are used suppositories

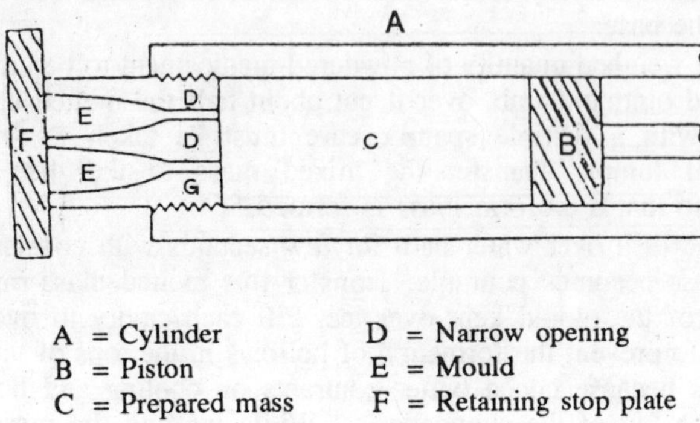

A = Cylinder
B = Piston
C = Prepared mass
D = Narrow opening
E = Mould
F = Retaining stop plate

Fig. 10.2 Cold compressing machine for suppositories.

should be separately wrapped in waxed paper or tin foil. Glycerogelatin suppositories should be packed in well closed glass or plastic containers.

Labelling

Suppositories should be labelled with the instructions "Store in a cool place." and warning "Not to be taken orally." or "For rectal use only.".

Rx

Alum 300 mg
Theobroma oil q.s.

Fiat : Suppositorium. Mitte tales quarta.
Sig : Unus omni nocte utendum.
Displacement value of alum is 2.0.

Procedure

To take into consideration the wastage calculate for five suppositories instead of four.

Melt the calculated quantity of theobroma oil in a dish over water bath. Pour about half of the melted theobroma oil on powdered alum already placed on a tile, mix thoroughly. Transfer the mixed mass to the dish, if necessary warm to make the mass pourable. Pour the melted mass into the cavities of the mould already lubricated and kept on ice. Fill five cavities to overflowing. Allow the mass to solidify. When the mass has solidified, trim off excess of the mass with a sharp blade or knife. Open the mould and remove the suppositories. If any lubricant is present wipe it off with filter paper or clean cloth. Wrap the suppositories individually in wax paper and then pack in partitioned cardboard boxes.

Uses

Alum suppositories are used as an astringent.

Rx

Hamamelis dry extract 200 mg
Theobroma oil q.s.

Fiat : Suppositorium. Mitte tales sex.
Signa : Unum nocte si opus sit utendum.
Displacement value of hamamelis dry extract is 1.5.

Procedure

To take into consideration the wastage calculate for eight suppositories instead of six.

Melt the calculated amount of theobroma oil in a dish over water bath. Pour about half of the melted theobroma oil on hamamelis dry extract already placed on a tile, mix thoroughly. Transfer the mixed mass to the dish, if necessary warm to make the mass pourable. Pour the melted mass into the cavities of the mould already lubricated and kept on ice. Fill five cavities to overflowing. Allow the mass to solidify. When the mass has solidified, trim off excess of the mass with a sharp blade or knife. Open the mould, remove the suppositories. If any lubricant is present, wipe it off with filter paper or clean cloth. Wrap the suppositories individually in wax paper and then pack in partitioned cardboard boxes.

Uses

These suppositories are used in the treatment of haemorrhoids.

Evaluation of Suppositories

Every batch of suppositories manufactured by moulding or by compression methods must be tested to ensure that the required standards are met or not. Each suppository must be visually examined for general appearance. The suppositories containing the medicaments in suspension form should be sliced longitudinally to determine uniform distribution of the medicament throughout the suppository. Assays for active medicaments must be carried out to ensure that they conform to labelled amounts of drugs or not.

The other tests which must be performed on suppositories include :

1. Uniformity of weight test.
2. Melting range test.
3. Liquefaction or softening time test.
4. Breaking test.
5. Disintegration/dissolution test.

1. Uniformity of Weight Test

All the suppositories should be uniform in weight. The weight variation may result if some cavities are underfilled and other are overfilled. To perform this test 20 suppositories are weighed and average weight is calculated. Then each suppository is weighed individually and weight noted. No suppository should deviate from the average weight by more than 5% except that two should not deviate by more than 7.5%.

2. Melting Range Test

This test is also known as macromelting range test. During this test the time taken for the entire suppository to melt is measured when immersed in a constant temperature, i.e., 37°C water bath. The apparatus used to perform this test is a USP tablet disintegration apparatus. The suppository is completely immersed in the constant water bath and the time for the whole suppository to melt or disperse in the surrounding water is noted. This test is performed for suppositories containing fatty base only to check the physical and absorption characteristics of each batch of suppositories.

3. Liquefaction or Softening Time Test

This test is performed on rectal suppositories to determine the softening time of the suppositories. During this test a glass rod is placed on the suppository held in U-tube of the apparatus immersed in constant temperature water bath. The time taken for the rod to pass through the suppository to the constriction of the apparatus is recorded as the softening time.

4. Breaking Test

Breaking or fragility tests are carried out to determine the tensile strength of the suppositories to assess whether they will be able to withstand the hazards of packing, transporting of normal handling or not.

5. Disintegration/Dissolution Test

The disintegration and dissolution times can be determined by using the same apparatus available for these tests on compressed tablets with necessary modifications in the test media. Suppositories prepared with water soluble bases are subjected to these tests.

Use of Suppositories for Drug Absorption

Generally the suppositories are used to produce local action at the site of application but many of them are also used to produce systemic effects. Drugs such as emollients, astringents, antibiotics, hormones, steroids and local anesthetics are formulated as suppositories for treating local conditions of rectum, vagina or urethra.

Rectal suppositories are mainly used for the treatment of constipation and haemorrhoids. Suppositories are also administered through the rectum to produce systemic action. A wide variety of drugs like analgesics, antispasmodics, sedatives, tranquilisers and antibiotics are used for this purpose. The drugs which irritate the gastrointestinal tract, cause vomitting, are destroyed by the hepatic circulation, or are destroyed in the stomach by pH changes, enzymes, etc., can be conveniently administered in the form of rectal suppositories.

Factors Affecting Drug Absorption from Rectal Suppositories

The rate of release and absorption of drugs from suppositories depends on the following factors :

1. Physiologic factors
2. Physico-chemical characteristics of the drug
3. Physico-chemical characteristics of the base and adjuvants.

1. Physiologic Factors

A number of drugs cannot be administered orally because either they get destroyed in the stomach by the digestive juices or their therapeutic activity is modified or reduced by the liver after absorption but if the same drug is administered through the rectum, the therapeutic value is retained because the drugs are directly absorbed into the blood circulation thus bypassing the liver. About 50 to 70% drugs administered through the rectum were reported to be absorbed directly into the general circulation.

The pH of the rectal fluids plays a significant role in the drug absorption. It was proved that weaker acids and bases are more readily absorbed than the stronger, highly ionized ones. As such change in pH of the rectal fluids is likely to enhance absorption rates of acidic and basic drugs. The absorption of acidic drugs was markedly increased when the pH of the surrounding fluids was decreased. The absorption of salicylic acid was increased from 12% at pH 7 to 42% at pH 4. Similarly in the case of quinine which is a basic drug the absorption was decreased from 20% at pH 7 to 9% at pH 4. This is due to the reason that quinine becomes more ionized at lower pH values.

The condition of the anorectal membrane also plays a role in the absorption of drugs. This membranous wall is covered with a continuous layer of mucous which can act as a mechanical barrier for the free passage of drug molecules through the pore space where absorption occurs.

2. Physico-Chemical Characteristics of the Drug

For the absorption of drugs it must first of all be released from the suppository and distributed by the surrounding fluids to the sites of absorption. If a drug is fat soluble the release to the aqueous fluids will be quite slow but if the drug is water soluble then it will be released at a faster rate. After the drug has been released it is distributed by the fluids to the sites of absorption. The distribution does not depend only on the nature of the drug but also depends on the presence or absence of surfactants and physiological conditions of the colon as well as the chemical nature of the solids and liquids present in it.

3. Physico-Chemical Characteristics of the Base and Adjuvants

Various physical and chemical properties of different suppository bases can affect absorption of drugs to a great extent. Absorption rate is faster from oily bases having lower melting points than from those having higher melting points. Since fatty bases may become hard after moulding, resulting in higher melting point which would affect the absorption.

Adjuvants included in the formulation of suppositories can affect dissolution of the drug in the fluids as well as absorption of drugs by changing the rheological characteristics of the base at body temperature.

In emulsion type suppository bases it was shown that the release of amount of water soluble drug was increased with the increase in water content of the base.

Though suppositories are considered as a good dosage form for the absorption of drugs but there are conflicting reports with respect to blood levels of drugs when administered in the form of suppositories. The information is difficult to correlate because of different or inadequate methods for determining blood levels, the nature of the drug and the suppository base as well as the inability of many patients to retain the suppository. Blood levels of theophylline derivatives were determined by its administration in the oral, intravenous and rectal dosage forms. Rectal retention enemas and intravenous injections showed comparable results if an allowance of 30 minutes delay is made in the rectal form.

Rectum or colon is considered as a dependable site for drug absorption but all the workers do not agree to it. A study for the absorption time on six drugs namely sodium salicylate, chloral hydrate, methylene blue, atropine, morphine and sodium iodide was carried out. It was found that the first five drugs are absorbed more quickly from the rectum and produce more therapeutic effective levels than the oral route. Whereas in the case of sodium iodide the absorption is slower by rectal route than by oral route but varies from person to person. On the whole it is generally agreed that suppositories produce therapeutically adequate blood levels.

Marketed Suppositories

1. Betadine vaginal pessaries (Win-Medicare Ltd., New Delhi - 110019).

   Contains :

   Povidone iodine 200 mg

2. Candid-V-1 tablets (Glenmark Pharmaceuticals Ltd., Bombay - 400026).

   Each contains :

   Clotrimazole 500 mg

3. Dulcolax suppositories (German Remedies Ltd., Bombay - 400018).

   Each contains :

Bisacodyl	5 mg (infants)
	10 mg (adults)

   Suppository base q.s.

4. Imidil vaginal tablets (Lyka Labs Ltd., Bombay - 400099).

   Each contains :

   Clotrimazole 100 mg, 200 mg, 500 mg.

5. Lotril pessary (Gufic Ltd., Bombay - 400057).

   Each contains :

   Cotrimoxazole 100 mg.

Revision Questions

I. Very short answer type questions

(A) Define the following :

(i) Suppositories
(ii) Suppository base
(iii) Pessaries
(iv) Displacement value
(v) Suppository mould

(B) Fill in the blanks :

(a) Suppositories are solid ...... dosage form of medicament.
(b) Suppositories are meant for ...... into the body cavities other than ......
(c) Cocoa butter is also known as ....
(d) Cocoa butter is not suitable base for the preparation of ...... and ...... bougies.
(e) Suppositories are prepared by three methods namely ......, ... and ...... method.

II. Short answer type questions

1. Write short notes on the following :
   (a) Uses of suppositories
   (b) Newer concept of suppositories
   (c) Displacement value
   (d) Glycerogelatin suppositories
   (e) Hot process or fusion method of preparation of suppositories
   (f) Advantage of synthetic bases over theobroma oil.
2. Differentiate between rectal suppositories and vaginal suppositories.
3. Explain the reasons :
   (i) Why the moulds require lubrication for oily or aqueous suppository bases?
   (ii) Why the synthetic suppository bases do not require lubrication of the moulds?
   (iii) Why the cotton wool should not be used for lubricating the moulds?
   (iv) Why is it necessary to take into consideration the displacement value of drugs in the preparation of suppositories?
   (v) Why the hydraulically operated cold-compression machines require cooling by water jackets?

III. Long answer type questions

1. What are suppositories? Describe advantages of suppositories and explain different types of suppositories.
2. Explain the term 'suppository base' Discuss various qualities of an ideal suppository base. Describe various types of bases used for the preparation of suppositories.
3. What is displacement value? Why is it necessary to take into consideration the displacement value of a drug? How will you determine the displacement value of the medicaments?
4. What are suppositories? Describe the methods of preparation of suppositories.
5. (a) Discuss various tests performed for the evaluation of suppositories.
   (b) Describe newer concept of suppositories.

11. Explain various factors affecting drug absorption from rectal suppositories.
12. Name at least three marketed suppositories.

Answers

I. B

(a) Unit
(b) Introduction, mouth
(c) Theobroma oil
(d) Pessaries, nasal
(e) Rolling, moulding, cold compression

11

Dental and Cosmetic Preparations

From time immemorial, people have used cosmetics to enhance their personal appeal by using different kinds of preparations. The cosmetics which are widely used now a days include tooth pastes, tooth powders, mouth washes, shampoos, nail polishes and polish removers, face powders, cold creams, vanishing creams and talcum powder, etc.

According to Drug and Cosmetics Act, the cosmetics are defined as the articles which are intended to be rubbed, poured, sprinkled, sprayed, introduced in, or otherwise applied to any part of the human body for cleansing, protecting, beautifying, promoting attractiveness or altering appearance.

A cosmetic only cleans, beautifies, alters the appearance, adds fragrance or stops the development of bad odour, it changes, increases or decreases the colour but it does not have any medicinal effect on the body. Thus ordinary toothpastes and toothpowders are cosmetics since they are used to clean the teeth and impart a pleasant feeling to the breath. But if such dentifrices include drugs such as antibiotics, fluorides, ammoniated materials and other substances which bring changes in the oral cavity then these preparations can be called drugs although they may not cease to be cosmetics.

Soap is used by almost everyone and is considered more of a bodily necessity than a cosmetic but toilet and bath soaps are specifically excluded from cosmetics. Similarly preparations such as room deodorants, etc., are not cosmetics but if the same deodorant is applied on the body it is termed as cosmetic. The devices or toilet articles used in applying the cosmetics such as tweezers, razor blades and combs should not be included in cosmetics.

Most cosmetics are safe for use by most people but adverse reactions occurs in many cosmetics such as deodorants/antiperspirants, hair removers, hair sprays, eye creams, hair colour/dye lighteners, facial skin creams/ cleansers and nail polishes.

The cosmetics are mostly used by women and they are more concerned about the chemical characteristics of cosmetics rather they are extremely concerned about the physical characteristics like texture, consistency, colour, odour, packaging and general appearance of cosmetics than chemical characteristics.

Classification of Cosmetics

Cosmetics are generally classified as follows :

(a) According to their functions
(b) According to their use
(c) According to their physical nature.

(a) According to their functions

(i) Decorative functions, e.g., nail polishes, eye lashes, lipstick, etc.
(ii) Corrective functions, e.g., dry creams and heavy face powders.
(iii) Protective functions, e.g., dry creams and heavy face powers.
(iv) Curative or therapeutic functions, e.g., antiperspirants and hair preparations.

(b) According to their use

(i) For the skin, e.g., powders, creams, lotions, deodorants, bath and cleansing preparations, make up, etc.
(ii) For the hair, e.g., shampoos, tonics, hair dressings, hair waving preparations, beard softeners, shaving preparations, hair removers (depilatories), etc.
(iii) For the nails, e.g., nail polish and polish removers, manicure preparations, etc.
(iv) For the teeth and mouth, e.g., dentifrices, mouth washes, etc.
(v) Borderline and kindred products, e.g., eye products, foot powders and applications, insect repellents, etc.

(c) According to their physical nature

(i) Aerosols, e.g., hair sets, perfumes, after-shave sprays, etc.
(ii) Cakes, e.g., rouge compacts, etc.
(iii) Emulsions, e.g., cold cream, vanishing cream, liquid cream, etc.
(iv) Jellies, e.g., hand jelly, wave set jelly, brilliantine jelly, etc.
(v) Mucilages, e.g., wave set, hand lotion, etc.
(vi) Oils, e.g., brilliantine, hair oils, etc.
(vii) Pastes, e.g., tooth paste, deodorant paste, etc.
(viii) Powders, e.g., face powder, tooth powder, talcum powder, etc.
(ix) Soaps, e.g., shampoo soap, shaving soap, toilet soap, etc.
(x) Solutions, e.g., after-shave lotions, hair sets, astringent lotions, etc.
(xi) Sticks, e.g., lipsticks, deodorant sticks, etc.
(xii) Suspensions, e.g., liquid powder, cosmetic stockings, etc.

In the manufacture of cosmetics all the raw materials used should be of highest quality and they should be standardised for their quality. All water used in cosmetic manufacture should be distilled or purified water. The colours used should be the permitted colours. The perfumes used should be compatible with other ingredients of the preparation.

New products should not be sent to the market immediately after their manufacture. They should be tested under all conditions particularly extremes of temperature and humidity conditions to which they are likely to encounter in the market. They should also be tested for shelf life by placing the product on the shelf for at least six months. If the sample passes all the tests then and only then it should be sent to the market.

1. Dentifrices

Dentifrices are the preparations meant to be applied to the teeth such as tooth paste and tooth powder. Generally they are applied with a tooth brush or fingers of the hand for cleaning the accessible surfaces of the teeth. They enhance the personal appearance of the teeth, reduce tooth decay and bad odour of the mouth and also make the gums healthy.

Now a days dentifrices have become very common and most people consider tooth paste or tooth powder a practical necessity. That is why the advertisers often promote such products with an eye to glamour and sex appeal. In recent years a number of dental products are developed which are capable of reducing tooth decay or diseases of the gums. The ingredients that are commonly used for such preparations include stannous fluoride and chlorophyll. It is claimed that when fluoride tooth paste is used regularly and at an early age, it reduces the incidence of tooth decay.

In the preparation of dentifrices the following ingredients are used :

(i) Polishing Agents (Abrasives)

Abrasives which are also known as polishing agents are used to remove debris and residual stains from the teeth and for polishing the tooth surface. They are white solid cleansing materials and constitute about half the total weight of the dental preparation. The commonly used abrasives include precipitated calcium carbonate, tribasic calcium phosphate, calcium pyrophosphate, hydrated alumina, magnesium trisilicate, etc.

(ii) Surface-Active Agents (Detergents)

Surface-active agents are added to enhance the action of polishing agents by wetting the teeth, the food particle, if any, and to emulsify the mucous. Examples are dioctyl sodium sulphosuccinate, sodium lauryl sulphate, etc. Soap can also be used for this purpose but to a lesser extent due to incompatibility with calcium salts and flavouring agents.

(iii) Humectant

A humectant is added to tooth paste which will keep it in the moist form and will not allow the paste to become dry. Moreover it will help in mixing the solid ingredients. The most commonly used humectants are glycerin, sorbitol and propylene glycol. Glycerin is sweet in taste and is regarded as the best humectant. It is added in the proportion of 5 to 10% by weight of the formulation.

(iv) Binders

A binder is added to keep the solids and liquids in the united form and also to maintain the consistency. The most commonly used binders are gum tragacanth, gum karaya, sodium alginate, methyl cellulose, etc. Gum tragacanth is generally used because it maintains the consistency, weather resistant and is not affected by pH changes. It is used in the proportion of 1 to 2.5%.

(v) Sweetening Agents

A sweetening agent is added to dentifrices to impart sweet taste to the preparation. It is generally added by blending with flavouring agents. Saccharin in the ratio of 0.005 to 0.25% is the most commonly used sweetening agent for this purpose.

(vi) Flavouring Agents

Flavouring agent is one of the most important ingredients of dentifrices and its selection is also very important because the choice of flavour varies from individual to individual. The most commonly used flavouring agents include peppermint, winter green, and cinnamon-mint, etc. The quantity of flavouring agent to be added depends on the type of flavour, type of the base and consumer acceptance. Generally it is used in the ratio of 0.5 to 2%.

(vii) Preservatives

The moisture and carbohydrates present in tooth paste lead to bacterial growth so a preservative should be included in the tooth paste to preserve its quality and stability. Generally methyl paraben and propyl paraben are used for this purpose. Sodium benzoate is not used as preservative in tooth pastes.

(viii) Therapeutic Agents

Therapeutic agents are included in medicated tooth pastes in order to check dental diseases and to remove bad smell but all tooth pastes do not contain these agents. The therapeutic agents which have bactericidal, bacteriostatic, enzyme inhibiting or acid neutralizing properties are used in medicated tooth pastes. The commonly used medicinal agents are fluorides, chlorophyll, urea, dibasic ammonium phosphate, sodium dehydroacetate, etc.

The dentifrices containing therapeutic agents should not be used daily, it may spoil the tooth structure.

Qualities of dentifrices

Tooth paste or tooth powder should have the following qualities :

1. When applied to the teeth it must remove foreign particles, food substances, plaque and clean the teeth.
2. It must be nontoxic.
3. It must be properly flavoured and sweetened.
4. It must leave the mouth with a refreshing after-taste.

Formulations for tooth paste and tooth powders

Formula No. 1 (Tooth paste)

Precipitated chalk, light	44.0 gm
Colloidal clay	3.0 gm
Tragacanth mucilage (2%)	3.0 gm
Glucose	4.0 gm
Glycerin	15.0 gm
Water	30.3 ml
Methyl paraben	0.2 gm
Peppermint oil	0.5 ml

Procedure

Warm the water in a dish. To this dissolve glucose; add glycerin and tragacanth mucilage. Separately pass precipitated chalk and colloidal clay through a fine sieve to remove the gritty particles. Incorporate these solids slowly to the liquids with continuous stirring until a smooth paste is obtained. Then add methyl paraben and peppermint oil, mix thoroughly until uniform. Pack in a suitable container.

Formula No. 2 (Tooth paste)

Dicalcium phosphate	35	gm
Calcium carbonate	14	gm
Glycerin	20	gm
Gum tragacanth	1.2	gm
Saccharin	50	mg
Sodium lauryl sulphate	10	gm
Water	19.8	ml

Flavour, sufficient quantity.

Procedure

Mix water and glycerin. To this add solid substances which have been passed through a sieve, with stirring. Then add flavour and mix thoroughly. Pack in a suitable container.

Formula No. 3 (Tooth powder)

Precipitated calcium carbonate	93.5	gm
Hard soap, powdered	50	gm
Saccharin	2	gm
Peppermint oil	4	ml
Cinnamon oil	2	ml
Methyl salicylate	7	ml

Procedure

Pass the solid substances through a fine sieve and mix them. To the mixed powders add the flavouring agents and mix thoroughly. Again pass through the siéve to remove the lumps, if formed.

Formula No. 4 (Tooth powder)

Precipitated calcium carbonate	150 gm
Magnesium carbonate	25 gm
Calcium peroxide	22 gm
Saccharin	100 mg
Flavour	3 ml

2. Facial Cosmetics

(i) Face Powder

Among all the cosmetics used, face powder undoubtedly leads the list. Face powder is not only used by women but men also use coloured face powder either after shave or to cover up the need of a shave temporarily.

A face powder is a cosmetic preparation which is applied to the face by means of a powder puff. It is generally applied at the end of the make up process, as a finishing touch.

In the preparation of face powder due consideration must be given to woman's requirement specially the odour and colour. The raw materials used should be of highest quality. The various raw materials used in the formulations of face powders include talc, kaolin, calcium carbonate, magnesium carbonate, zinc stearate, magnesium stearate, calcium silicate, colour and perfume.

Characteristics of a face powder

A face powder should have the following properties :

(i) It should be very fine and should not have any gritty particle.
(ii) The ingredients should be evenly distributed.
(iii) It should be non-toxic and non-irritant to the skin.
(iv) It should be chemically and physically stable.
(v) It should spread easily and adhere to the skin.
(vi) It should have good absorbing property.

(vii) It should remove shine from the face.

(viii) It should cover minor imperfections of the face and should not appear as paint.

(ix) It should look natural.

(x) It should not dust off in a few minutes and make repowdering necessary.

Formulations for face powder

Formula No. 1

Kaolin	10 gm
Light calcium carbonate	15 gm
Zinc oxide	15 gm
Zinc stearate	5 gm
Magnesium carbonate	5 gm
Talc	50 gm

Perfume, sufficient quantity.

Formula No. 2 (Baby powder)

Talc	85	gm
Zinc stearate	10	gm
Boric acid	4.75	gm
Perfume	0.25	ml

Formula No. 3 (Deodorant powder)

Boric acid	5 gm
Salicylic acid	3 gm
Starch	50 gm
Talc	42 gm

Method of preparation

For the preparation of above mentioned powders all the ingredients should be mixed thoroughly and passed through sieve no. 120 to get a very fine powder. The powder so produced should be packaged in a powder box of highest quality which should be odorless under normal conditions of use and storage.

(ii) Compact Powder

A compact powder is simply a face powder which is pressed in the form of a cake and is applied on the face with a powder puff. A large volume of the powder is reduced by compression into a shallow metal container known as plate or compressed directly into the container. The formulation is so adjusted that the cake will not break after compression or during use.

Formula for compact powder

Talc	50 gm
Zinc oxide	10 gm
Kaolin	15 gm
Titanium dioxide	5 gm
Calcium carbonate	15 gm
Rice starch	5 gm
Binder solution	5 ml
Perfume, sufficient quantity.	

Formula for binder solution

Gum tragacanth	2 gm
Glucose	5 gm
Water	93 ml
Preservatives, sufficient quantity.	

Procedure

Mix the solid ingredients which have already been passed through sieve no. 120. To the mixed powders add the binding solution and perfume. Mix thoroughly so as to get a wet mass of desired consistency. Compress the mass and dry the cake. The compact must neither be too hard nor too soft. The powder must come off easily on the puff and the cake must not get hard.

Marketed Compact Powders

1. Lakme
2. Gala of London
3. Clear Touch
4. Ravon 2-way cake.
5. Tips & Toes.

(iii) Rouges

A rouge is a preparation which is applied to the cheeks for enhancing the face beauty and to impart and stimulate the rosy freshness of the young and healthy skin. It is very commonly applied by the smartly turned out women. A rouge is a very important item in a ladies set of cosmetics. Without the inclusion of a rouge the cosmetic set for ladies is incomplete.

Various types of rouges such as liquid, cream and solid rouges are available in numerous shades. Solid rouges are stable and easy to apply. Dry compact rouge is applied by means of a puff.

Formula for dry rouge

Talc	4.8 gm
Kaolin	1.6 gm
Chalk	0.4 gm
Magnesium carbonate	0.4 gm
Zinc stearate	0.4 gm
Titanium dioxide	1.2 gm
Colour	1.2 gm
Perfume, sufficient quantity.	

Method of preparation

All the ingredients are mixed thoroughly so as to distribute the colour uniformly. The mixed powder is molded by hand or by automatic machine. Then the molded mass is pressed to expel the air from the interstices of powder particles. After the compacts have been formed they are dried at a uniformly slow rate of temperature to avoid a dry mist and an undesirable top cast.

(iv) Cold Creams

Cold creams are the cosmetic preparations which are applied on the face. The name cold cream is given because of cooling effect of such products on the skin. They are generally prepared by emulsification of oils and water. Beeswax-borax cleansing cream is the most widely used cream.

Formula for beeswax-borax cleansing cream

Bees wax	4.0 gm
Liquid paraffin	39.8 gm
White soft paraffin	12.0 gm
Hard paraffin	12.0 gm
Borax	0.2 gm
Water	32.0 ml
Perfume, sufficient quantity.	

Formula for cold cream

White bees wax	7.3 gm
Stearic acid	13.6 gm
Wool fat	9.0 gm
Liquid paraffin	15.0 gm
Terpineol	1.5 gm
Triethanolamine	1.9 gm
Propylene glycol	7.3 gm
Water	43.2 gm
Perfume, sufficient quantity.	

Procedure

Melt stearic acid, white bees wax, and wool fat on water bath. Then add terpineol. Separately warm water to almost same temperature as that of melted oils and add triethanolamine. Incorporate warmed aqueous liquid to the melted oils and stir continuously so as to get a creamy emulsion. Then add propylene glycol in which perfume has been mixed. Stir thoroughly until a smooth cream is formed and it cools down to room temperature.

Marketed Cold Creams

1. Lakme
2. Ponds
3. Nivea
4. Charmis
5. Emami
6. Johnson's baby cream.

(v) Vanishing Creams

Vanishing creams are oil-in-water type emulsions which are prepared by emulsification of stearic acid and water by means of alkalies such as sodium hydroxide, potassium hydroxide, borax triethanolamine, etc. Glycerin is also added. Stearic acid is the most important constituent of vanishing creams hence a good quality triple pressed stearic acid should be selected.

Formula for vanishing cream

Stearic acid	18.8 gm
Glycerin	2.7 gm
Lanolin	2.0 gm
Triethanolamine	1.0 gm
Water	80.0 ml
Preservative	1.0 gm

Perfume, sufficient quantity.

Procedure

Melt stearic acid and lanolin. Separately mix water, glycerin and triethanolamine and warm to almost the same temperature as that of melted substances. Mix the two with continuous stirring. Add the preservative and perfume. Mix thoroughly until a uniform product is obtained.

(vi) Preparations for Eye Make-up

(a) Eye Shadow

Eye shadow is used to give a background of colour to the eyes and is applied to the eye lids. There are a large number of shades which are used but more commonly used are blue, green, grey, white, gold and silver colourings. Eye shadows are prepared in wax bases in the form of creams, emulsions, sticks, loose powders or as compressed powders.

(b) Eyebrow Pencils

Eyebrow pencils are hard crayons, usually black and are used for darkening the eyebrows. These are manufactured by the pencil manufacturers and are available in wide range of colours. The eyebrow pencils contain a high proportion of waxes to make them hard so that they can be molded as a thin stick and sharpened to a point.

(c) Mascara

Mascara is a dark pigmented preparation used on the eyelashes and eyebrows to darken and thicken their appearance. It is applied with a brush.

In the preparation of mascara special care must be taken in the selection of colour and other ingredients. Mascara should have the following qualities :

(i) It must be non-toxic.
(ii) It must be non-irritating to the eyes.
(iii) It must not run, cake or cause eyelashes to stick together.
(iv) It should be applied easily and evenly.

(vii) Lipsticks

Lipstick is the most widely used item of cosmetics by the women to brighten the colour of the lips. Without the inclusion of lipsticks in the bag of cosmetics of an Indian woman it is considered as incomplete bag. Lipsticks are usually manufactured as molded sticks and basically consist of colouring pigments dissolved or dispersed in a fatty base which is made stiff by including wax so as to form a stick. Suitable perfumes and flavours are also incorporated. Depending on the cost of raw materials used in the manufacture of lipsticks they are available in cheap and costlier varieties and in different shades. A good quality lipstick should have the following qualities :

1. It should be non-toxic and non-irritating.
2. It should be free from gritty particles.
3. It should be easily applicable and easily removable if need arises.
4. It should have good odour.
5. It should give shiny and smooth appearance.
6. It should not dry on storage.
7. It should be free from sweating.
8. It should maintain its lip colour long after its application.
9. The stick should not break during use and it should maintain its firmness till whole of it is used up.

Formula for lipsticks

Beeswax, white	33.0 gm
Cetyl alcohol	12.0 gm
Seasame oil	20.0 ml
Castor oil	29.0 gm
Perfume	2.0 ml
Tetrabromfluorescein	4.0 gm

Procedure

Dissolve tetrabromfluorescein in castor oil. Melt beeswax, cetyl alcohol, and seasame oil together. Mix the two solutions and add perfume. Mix thoroughly so as to get a uniform mass. Transfer the mass so prepared into the cavities of the molds.

(viii) Shaving Media

Shaving media are really not the cosmetics for the hair but they are used to remove unsightly hair particularly from men's faces. Women also use them in limited amounts to remove hair from legs, under the arm and other conspicuous places with or without the help of a razor.

Various types of shaving media include :

(a) Preshave products, e.g., beard softeners and pre electric shaving lotions.

(b) Shaving products include brushless shaving creams, lather shaving creams and shaving soaps. Shaving soaps are employed as cakes, sticks, powders, creams and liquids in wooden or plastic bowls of various designs and sizes. For a long time soaps were quite commonly used as a shaving media but now a days they are largely replaced with brushless and lather shaving creams.

(c) After shave products include lotions and gels used to refresh the skin after shave.

Lather Shaving Creams

Lather shaving creams are semisolid preparations which are used by men to help in removing the hair from the face. These creams are packaged in collapsible tubes and are used with the help of shaving brush to produce a lather on the face thus soften the beard and hold individual hair erect for close shaving. They also provide lubricity for the razor, making the shaving process smooth and comfortable.

Lather shaving creams are generally formulated as heavy, concentrated (40 to 60%) soap solutions in glycerol and water. The soap is formed by the saponification of fatty acids and oils with alkalies. Glycerin is extensively used as humectant in these types of shaving creams. The ingredients commonly used in the preparation of shaving creams include stearic acid, tallow, stearin, coconut oil, olive oil, peanut oil, caustic soda, caustic potash, glycerin, alcohol, lanolin, borax, boric acid, propylene glycol, aromatic water and water. Colouring and flavouring agents may be added according to choice and depending on the nature of other ingredients.

Qualities of a good lather shaving cream

A good lather shaving cream should have the following qualities :

1. It should be non-irritating to the skin.
2. It should not change its viscosity according to temperature.
3. It should be smooth, soft and non-lumpy.
4. It should have good wetting properties.
5. It must produce rich lather composed of small bubbles that do not dry on the face too rapidly.
6. Only small quantity of cream should be required to produce good lather, i.e., it should be economical.
7. It should be non-corrosive to the razor blade and easily rinsed from the razor and face.

Formula for lather shaving cream

Stearic acid	38.8 gm
Coconut oil	9.7 gm
Potassium hydroxide	8.0 gm
Sodium hydroxide	1.6 gm
Glycerol	11.6 gm
Water	30.3 ml

Preservative, sufficient quantity.
Perfume, sufficient quantity.

Method of preparation

Melt half of the stearic acid with coconut oil over water bath. To this add alkalies with continuous stirring to saponify the oils. After saponification add the remainder of stearic acid. Separately warm the glycerol and half of water to about 65°C and add slowly to the saponified liquid with continuous stirring until a creamy paste is formed. Heat the remaining amount of water to about 44°C and add quickly to the cream with continuous stirring. Add the preservative and perfume, stir so as to mix thoroughly.

3. Antiperspirants and Deodorants

Bad odour emitted by the body of both men and women is a great problem. Women are more peculiar about it. So the substances which are used to overcome this bad smell are known as antiperspirants and deodorants. The sweat glands secrete perspiration which varies from person to person. Some individuals secrete sweat which is of offensive odour and in certain cases it is considerably coloured. The correction of body odour is carried out by antiperspirants and deodorants.

Antiperspirants and deodorant are cosmetic products which are used to reduce underarm and body odour. Antiperspirants inhibit the flow of perspiration and deodorants inhibit the formation of malodour in perspiration by suppressing bacterial growth or cover the malodour with a more pleasing one. Many products have both antiperspirant and deodorant action.

Antiperspirants contain substances which have astringent action and react with proteins of the skin, causing coagulation accompanied by a swelling at the opening of the sweat glands thus blocking the openings and reducing the flow of sweat. Antiperspirants and deodorants are available as clear liquids for direct, spray or aerosol application, powder sprays, sticks, creams and lotions.

Salts of various metals such as aluminium, iron, chromium, lead, mercury, zinc and zirconium have astringent properties which precipitate the proteins but all of them cannot be used because of either discolouration or toxic effects but salts of ammonium and zinc are most commonly used. To protect the skin from toxic effects and cloths from rotting a combination of salts may be used. The liquid antiperspirants consist of an aqueous or hydroalcoholic solution of an astringent salt to which a small amount of humectant, a perfume, a dispersing agent for the perfume and a deodorant is added.

Formula for deodorant powder

Salicylic acid	2.0 gm
Boric acid	40.0 gm
Talc	48.0 gm
Zinc stearate	10.0 gm

Formula for liquid antiperspirant

Alcohol	50.0 ml
Propylene glycol	5.0 ml
Hexachlorophene	0.1 gm
Aluminium chlorohydroxide	15.0 gm
Water	29.9 ml

Perfume, sufficient quantity.

Method of preparation

Mix alcohol and propylene glycol. To this dissolve hexachlorophene and perfume. Separately dissolve aluminium chlorohydroxide in water. Add this solution slowly to the alcoholic solution. Keep the mixed solutions in a closed container for at least 48 hours, then filter the solution and fill in suitable containers.

4. Shampoos

A shampoo may be defined as a preparation containing surface active agents which when used will remove grease, dirt and debris from the hair and scalp without seriously affecting the hair, scalp and other parts of the body.

Apart from cleansing action it must leave the hair fragrant, lustrous, soft and manageable. Though the shampoos act as detergents like that of detergent cakes but along with these properties they behave as cosmetics.

Generally shampoos are water soluble solutions or suspensions prepared by dissolving cleansing agents in a suitable liquid to which other agents are added to improve the functions of the shampoo. Mostly synthetic detergents are used for this purpose to which soap is also added but good shampoos do not contain any soap.

Properties of a shampoo

A good shampoo should have the following qualities :

1. It should be effective in small amounts.
2. It should remove grease, dirt and skin debris from the hair and scalp.
3. It should be non-toxic, non-irritant and should not damage the skin and sensitive organs like eyes if accidentally comes in contact with the eyes.
4. It should produce adequate foam in soft as well as hard water.
5. It should give pleasant flavour after its use.
6. It should be easily washable with water.
7. It should leave the hair lustrous, soft and manageable.

Since time immemorial both men and women have used different types of preparations for cleaning their hair. Now a days it has become essential socially and personally for men and women to keep their hair healthy looking and aesthetically pleasing because good looking and properly dressed hair add to one's beauty and charming personality, specially to the women. Therefore, shampoos are widely used for this purpose which are available in different forms as described below :

1. Clear liquid shampoos
2. Baby shampoos
3. Medicated dandruff shampoos
4. Soap shampoos
6. Liquid cream or lotion shampoos
7. Powder shampoos
8. Gel shampoos
9. Cream or paste shampoos.

Various types of additives used in shampoos include :

1. Opacifiers

Opacifiers are used to make the shampoo opaque. Such substances include esters such as glycol and glyceryl stearate and higher alcohols such as cetyl and stearyl alcohol, stearate soaps and waxy alkylamides such as stearic amides.

2. Solubilizing Agents

Solubilizing agents are used to solubilize poorly soluble substances so as to get a clear shampoo. Solubilizing agents used include ethyl alcohol, glycerol, propylene glycol and diethylene glycol monoethyl ether. Surfactants are also used as solubilizing agents.

3. Thickening Agents

Thickening agents are used to increase the viscosity of the shampoos and provide the desired consistency to the preparation. Sodium stearate and stearic amides are excellent thickening agents for cream type shampoos. Polyvinyl alcohol, methyl cellulose and sodium alginate are also used for this purpose.

4. Conditioning Agents

Conditioning agents are used to improve the manageability and the texture of the hair. Various oils, fatty alcohols, glycol esters, humectants and protein derivatives are used for this purpose. Lanolin and its derivatives are also extensively used as hair conditioners. Certain surfactants are also used as hair conditioners.

5. Preservatives

Shampoos prepared with surfactants must be suitably preserved because such preparations lead to bacterial and mold growth. Methyl paraben and propyl paraben are commonly used preservatives in shampoos.

Formula for coconut oil shampoo

Coconut oil	37.0 gm
Potassium hydroxide	29.0 gm
Water	5.0 ml
Glycerin	29.0 gm
Perfume, sufficient quantity.	

Formula for cream type shampoo

Sodium lauryl sulphate	25.0	gm
Stearic acid	6.5	gm
Lanolin	0.25	gm

Caustic soda	1.0	gm
Cetyl alcohol	0.5	gm
Water	67.25	ml

Colouring agent, sufficient.
Perfume, sufficient.

Method of preparation

Dissolve cetyl alcohol, sodium lauryl sulphate, stearic acid and lanolin in about 80% water by heating in a water bath. Separately dissolve caustic soda in remaining amount of water and heat almost to the same temperature as the previous one. Then mix the two solutions with stirring. When the solution cools down add the colouring agent and perfume. Mix thoroughly so as to get a homogeneous product.

Marketed Shampoos

1. Clinic
2. Sunsilk
3. Park Avenue Bear shampoo
4. Lakme
5. Ultra Doux
6. Hallo

5. Hair Dressings

Since time immemorial hair dressings were used by men and women to impart good appearance to the hair. The products used for this purpose were home made commonly prepared with wines, herbs, animal and plant bi-products but now a days along with home made products newer products with good results are introduced in the market the demand of which is increasing day by day. Hair not only acts as a protective covering for the head but is also an attractive feature of men and women. Both of these factors, i.e., protection and attraction are best provided by healthy hair.

Characteristics of a good hair dressing

A good hair dressing preparation should have the following qualities :

1. It should have good grooming action.
2. It should provide lustre to the hair without greasiness.
3. It should be non-toxic to the skin.
4. It should provide some degree of hair conditioning.
5. It should provide anti-dandruff action.
6. It should have good wetting action.

The other preparations used for the hair include :

(i) Brilliantines

Brilliantines are used to impart lustre to the hair and also for keeping the hair in place. Liquid brilliantines are sprayed on the hair with an atomizer after the hair has been waved. The liquid type brilliantines are more commonly used by the women because they are easy to apply and more viscous types are preferred by the men.

(ii) Hair Conditioners

Hair conditioners are used to make the hair manageable, glossy and of soft texture. They are generally used for those hair which are damaged by too frequent shampooing, hair straighteners, bleaching and dyeing.

Hair rinses are applied to the hair after shampooing which will help to remove the detergent film that shampoo may leave. After rinsing they leave the hair too soft to touch. Cream rinses may contain proteins, antidandruff compounds and temporary dyes.

(iii) Hair Tonics

Hair tonics are the preparations which are applied to the hair for curing baldness, relieving oily or dry skin and to prevent or cure dandruff. Hair tonics generally contain a combination of at least two of the three ingredients, i.e., sebaceous gland stimulant, a rubefacient and an antiseptic.

Hair tonics should be rubbed into the scalp at night which should be shampooed out in the morning. It must be stated on the label of such preparations that longer the preparation is left on the scalp better would be the results.

(iv) Hair-Waving and Hair-Straightening Preparations

Since long men and women had a quest to beautify their hair by one way or the other. It has been observed that the individual with straight hair wants curly hair and the individual with curly hair believes that straight hair are more beautiful. Therefore both types, i.e., hair waving and straightening products are prepared.

In the olden days the home curling iron was most commonly used by women to make their hair curly and it is still used to a large extent. The curl produced by this method is temporary so improved methods are developed to produce better curls. The home hair curling procedures are used by special devices like curling irons, bobby pins and even fingers by which a finger wave is made. To help these more simple waving operations hair waving liquids are available under the name 'wave sets'. These solutions generally consist of thick colloidal solutions of gum karaya, gum acacia, gum tragacanth, gelatin, Irish moss or algin usually with the addition of alkali carbonates or borax, sulphonated oil, certain amine bases, sometimes shellac, glycerin, glycols or alcohol.

The method of preparation is quite simple. The gum is soaked in water overnight, next day it is heated to almost boiling and strained to get the mucilage. Cool to room temperature and add the other ingredients either directly or previously dissolved in water. Allow the preparations to stand for about three days to observe any change in viscosity. The viscosity of the preparation should not be changed during shelf-life. As there are chances of bacterial growth so a suitable preservative must be added.

Formula for hair wave set

Gum tragacanth ribbons	12.0 gm
Warm water	1.5 litres
Alcohol	160.0 ml
Perfume	4.0 ml
Sodium benzoate	1.0 gm

Method of preparation

Dissolve sodium benzoate in warm water and add gum tragacanth. Allow to stand overnight with occasional stirring. Then pass the solution through cheese cloth so as to remove lumps. Dissolve perfume in alcohol and add to the tragacanth solution; add the colour and mix thoroughly so as to get a homogeneous product.

The viscosity of the preparation can be adjusted by increasing or decreasing the quantity of water used.

Hair straightening products are closely related to hair waving products. Almost same process is used to straighten the hair as is used to curl it. Hair waving is generally done by chemical means whereas hair straightening is done by physical means which is more useful. In this method the hair is washed and dried thoroughly. Then the pressed oils are applied hot while the hair is being combed or stretched straight. Pressing oils generally contain waxes, perfume, lanolin and other hair conditioners in a petrolatum base.

(v) Hair Dyes

Since time immemorial both men and women used to dye their hair to change the natural colour, to colour the grey or white hair which has changed with age so as to restore a youthful appearance or to alter the colour of the hair temporarily for a particular occasion. Hair dyes are classified according to the duration of action as temporary, semipermanent or permanent dyes. Similarly the colouring products are classified as follows :

(i) Bleaching agents
(ii) Temporary colouring agents
(iii) Permanent colouring agents
(iv) Natural organic dyes.

Hair colouring products include dye containing creams, shampoos or rinses prepared by using substances obtained from plants, metallic compounds and mixture of these two types of substances. The most commonly used organic material from plant origin is 'Henna'.

Characteristics of a hair dye

An ideal hair dye should have the following characteristics :

(i) It should be non-irritating to the hair and skin.
(ii) It should be non-toxic.
(iii) It should be able to colour the hair shaft without damaging it.
(iv) It should be stable and should not change its colour when exposed to air, sunlight, water, shampoo or hair conditioning agents.

Marketed Hair Dyes

1. Godrej permanent liquid hair dye
2. Kesh kala hair darkner
3. Tru-tone gel
4. Wondrex cream hair dye
5. Bigen hair dye.

(vi) Depilatories (Hair Removers)

Depilatory products are used to soften unsightly human hair so that it can be easily removed by wiping or rinsing a short time after application. When the hair are removed by chemical methods it is known as depilation and when the relatively intact unwanted hair are removed by plucking, electrolysis and x-ray, etc., it is known as epilation.

Present day fashions in women have created a great demand for depilatories and it has been confirmed through market surveys that a large number of women population in the country remove superfluous hair either by mechanical or chemical methods. Women do not wish to appear mannish by having hair prominent, particularly on the face. They want to keep the legs, arms and armpits free from unsightly hair the year around if they are to wear sleeveless gowns, bathing suits and casual wears without embarrassment.

Though shaving is done biweekly by a few women but it is not a convenient method of removing the hair as it is not possible to shave all the parts of the body moreover it may lead to cuts and scratches. Therefore the use of depilatories has increased to a great extent. Such preparations are available as solids, semisolids as cream form or waxy preparations.

The chemicals most commonly used for the preparation of depilatories include metallic sulphides of barium, calcium and strontium. Other chemicals like tin salts, calcium thioglycerol and calcium thioglycollate are also used. Out of all these chemicals barium sulphide is the most popular depilating agent because it has excellent depilating properties without serious effects. When depilatories are applied to the skin they produce unpleasant odour and it is difficult to obtain a perfume which will be of value. The perfume materials include aromatic alcohols, ketones, ionones, anise, safrol and rose.

Qualities of a good depilatory

An ideal chemical depilatory should have the following qualities :

1. It should complete its action within 2-5 minutes and during this period it should make the hair soft, swelled and dispersed which should be removed from the skin by wiping or rinsing.
2. It should be non-toxic and non-irritant to the skin.
3. It should be easy to apply.
4. It should be economical to use.
5. It should be elegant, odourless or pleasantly flavoured.
6. It should remain stable in the container.

Formula for powder depilatory

Barium sulphide	31.0	gm
Titanium dioxide	18.0	gm
Maize starch	50.0	gm
Menthol	0.20	gm
Perfume	0.80	ml

Note : Mix with water at the time of application.

Formula for paste depilatory

Barium sulphide	8.0 gm
Calcium carbonate	32.0 gm
Powdered soap	4.0 gm
Glycerin	2.0 gm
Water	54.0 ml

Perfume, sufficient quantity.

Procedure

Dissolve powdered soap in water. To this add glycerin and mix. To this solution add barium sulphide and calcium carbonate which has been passed through a fine sieve. Mix and incorporate perfume with thorough trituration so as to get a smooth paste.

Marketed Hair Removers

1. Anne French
2. Lakme.

(vii) Antidandruff Preparations

Dandruff is a scaly disease of the scalp. A product which clears the scalp of adherent debris and regulates the amount of residual scalp and hair oils to retain healthy condition of the scalp is known as antidandruff preparation.

The sebaceous glands surround the hair and secrete their oil along the shaft of the hair. At times this oily secretion is mixed with decomposition matter from the cells which is horn like in nature and is forced to the surface of the scalp. The secretion may be deficient or excessive. If hygienic care of the scalp is not taken it may result in bacterial growth. The infection may result from barber shops, hat shops, public room or by using common comb.

Dandruff may lead to loss of hair but the exact reason for this is not known. Dandruff can be checked but not remedied by shampooing. Proper cleansing of the scalp is of great importance. This should be combined with treatments designed to reduce or stimulate the secretions of the sebaceous glands. Application of germicide is also helpful. Mechanical massage or thorough brushing of the hair with a clean brush both before and after the shampoo is advisable. The frequency of washing the hair is very important. If large quantity of dandruff is present, hair should be washed daily with a shampoo for about a week. If the dandruff is reduced the washing may be done after two or three days. While using shampoo preferably it should be allowed to remain on the hair for a quarter to half an hour which is then washed with warm water. After complete drying of the hair it should be massaged and brushed thoroughly to increase the blood supply. Various types of shampoos are available as antidandruff preparations.

Formula for antidandruff preparation

Selenium disulphide	2.5 gm
Surfactant	17.0 gm
Inert stabilizer	5.2 gm
Water	75.3 ml

Formula for loose dandruff remover

Betanaphthol	1.0 gm
Alcohol	48.9 ml
Tr. of quillaia	48.0 ml
Glycerin	2.0 ml
Perfume	0.1 ml

Revision Questions

I. Very short answer type questions

(A) Define the following :

(i) Cosmetics
(ii) Dentifrices
(iii) Face powders
(iv) Compact powders
(v) Rouges
(vi) Cold creams
(vii) Eye shadow
(viii) Mascara
(ix) Lipsticks
(x) Lather shaving creams
(xi) Antiperspirants
(xii) Deodorants
(xiii) Brilliantines
(xiii) Shampoos
(xiv) Hair tonics
(xv) Hair dyes
(xvi) Depilatories
(xvii) Anti-dandruff preparations.

(B) Fill in the blanks :

(a) Toilet and bath soaps are specifically ...... from cosmetics.
(b) Generally dentifrices are applied to the teeth with the help of ...... or ....
(c) The soap in lather shaving creams is formed by the ...... of fatty acids and oils with ....
(d) The perspiration is secreted by ....
(e) Dandruff leads to loss of ....

II. Short answer type questions

1. Write shorts notes on the following :
   (a) Dentifrices
   (b) Face powders
   (c) Cold creams
   (d) Lipsticks
   (e) Shampoos
   (f) Hair dyes
   (g) Antidandruff preparations
2. Give a suitable formula and method of preparation for toothpaste.
3. What are lather shaving creams give the qualities of a good lather shaving cream.
4. Describe the qualities of good face powders.
5. Explain the qualities of a good lipstick.
6. Name different types of hairdressings used. Give a brief account of hair waving and straightening preparations.
7. Give at least three examples of marketed preparations of the following :
   (a) Compact powders
   (b) Cold creams
   (c) Shampoos
   (d) Hair dyes

III. Long answer type questions

1. What are cosmetic preparations? Classify them. Describe face powders in brief.
2. What are dentifrices? What should be the qualities of dentifrices? Describe the formulation of dentifrices and give a suitable formula for tooth powder.
3. What are cold creams? How do they differ from vanishing creams? Give a suitable formula and method of preparation of a cold cream.
4. (a) What do you know about 'Lipsticks'? Explain the qualities of a good lipstick.

   (b) Discuss what you know about 'shaving media'.
5. What are shampoos? Describe the properties of a good shampoo and types of shampoos. Explain various types of additives used in the preparation of shampoos. Give a formula of a good shampoo.
6. Name the preparations used for hair dressing. Explain the characteristics of a good hairdressing and discuss hair dyes in detail.
7. What are 'depilatories'? Discuss different methods used for removing unwanted hair from the body. Explain the qualities and suitable formula for a good depilatory.
8. Explain antidandruff preparations. How the dandruff is produced and how antidandruff preparations help to check dandruff?
9. Differentiate between the following :
   (i) Rouges and compact face powder.
   (ii) Cold cream and vanishing cream
   (iii) Hair tonics and hair conditioners.
   (iv) Antiperspirants & deodorants.

Answers

I. (B)

(a) Excluded
(b) Brush, fingers
(c) Saponification, alkalies
(d) Sweat glands
(e) Hair

12

Parenteral Preparations

Parenteral preparations or injectables are the sterile solutions or suspensions of drugs in aqueous or oily vehicles meant for introduction into the body by means of an injection under or through one or more layers of the skin or mucous membrane. Since they are introduced into internal body compartments they must be sterile and free from all types of living microorganisms and microbial products such as toxins, pyrogens, etc., and should be free from particles like dust, fibres, etc. They should be isotonic with body fluids. An utmost care must be taken in the preparation of injectables to avoid all types of physical, chemical or microbial contaminations.

Parenteral preparations must be introduced through the same route for which they are intended, for example, if an oily suspension meant for intramuscular injection is introduced by intravenous injection may prove fatal. Similarly potent drugs meant for administration through intramuscular injection may lead to even death if given by intravenous injection.

ROUTES OF ADMINISTRATION OF PARENTERAL PRODUCTS

Various routes of administration of parenteral products are as follows :

1. Intracutaneous or Intradermal Injections

These injections ar given in between dermis and epidermis. Skin of the left forearm is usually selected for giving the injection. Absorption by this route is slow therefore usually small volume from 0.1 to 0.2 ml is injected. This route is mainly used for testing the sensitivity of the injectables and for diagnostic purposes.

2. Subcutaneous or Hypodermic Injections

These injections are given in the subcutaneous tissue under the skin of the upper arm. The volume of 1 ml or less can be injected by this route. This is the most popular route because it is convenient for the patient and the doctor.

3. Intramuscular Injections

These injections are given into the muscular tissues. The muscles of the

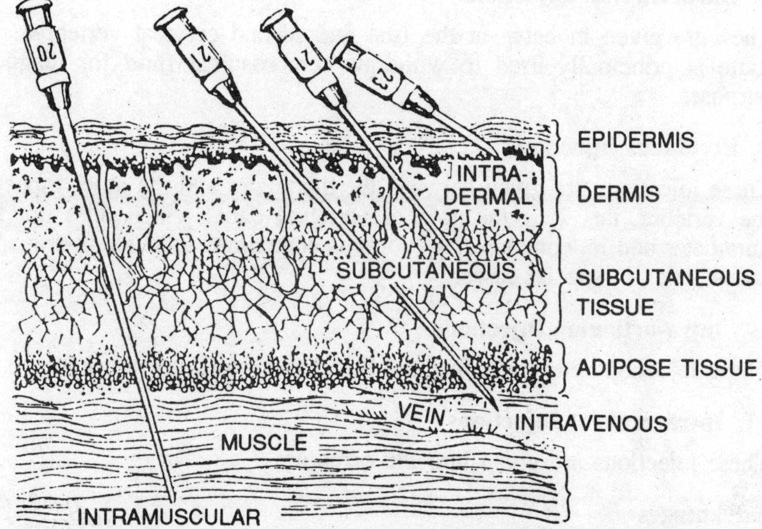

Fig. 12.1 Routes of administration of parenteral products.

shoulder, thigh or buttock are usually selected. Generally volume up to 2 ml is administered by this route and should not exceed 4 ml at one site.

4. Intravenous Injections

These injections are given into the vein therefore directly reach the blood stream. The median basilic vein which is near the elbow is usually selected because it is easily located and connects with the other major veins of the arm. Large volumes of solutions ranging from 1 ml to 500 ml or even more can be injected but volumes of more than 15 ml should be isotonic with blood. Oily injections and suspensions cannot be injected by this route.

5. Intra-arterial Injections

These injections are given directly into the artery when an immediate effect in a peripheral area is required. They are occasionally used.

Less Commonly Used Routes

6. Intracardiac Injections

They are given directly into the heart muscles or ventricle and are used in emergency only.

7. Intrathecal Injections

They are given into the subarachnoid space surrounding the spinal cord. This route is used for giving spinal anaesthesia.

8. Intracisternal Injections

They are given in between the first and second cervical vertebrae. This route is principally used to withdraw cerebrospinal fluid for diagnostic purposes.

9. Peridural Injections

These injections are given between the duramater and the inner aspects of the vertebra, i.e., it is the area of vertebral canal which does not have duramater and its contents. This route is sometimes used for giving spinal anaesthetics in special cases.

10. Intra-articular Injections

These injections are given into the liquid that lubricates the joints.

11. Intracerebral Injections

These injections are given into the cerebrum.

Advantages

1. Parenteral route of administration is used when a rapid onset of action of the drug is required, hence the route is used in emergency cases.
2. This route is preferred when the drugs are inactivated in the G.I.T. or drugs are not well absorbed after oral administration.
3. This is the most suitable route of administration of drugs in treating patients who are non-cooperative, unconscious or are otherwise unable to take the medicine orally.
4. Prolonged action of a drug can be successfully produced by this route.
5. Solutions in volumes from fraction of millilitre to 4 litres can be introduced by parenteral route.

Disadvantages

1. This mode of treatment is more expensive because it requires a technical and trained person for administration.
2. Sterilization is of utmost importance.
3. The administration of drug through wrong route of injection may prove fatal.
4. Daily or frequent administration of injections may pose difficulties to the patient.

TYPES OF PARENTERAL PREPARATIONS

Parenteral preparations may be classified as follows :

1. Solutions ready for injection.
2. Suspensions ready for injection.

3. Emulsions suitable for parenteral administration.
4. Dry, soluble products which are dissolved in a suitable solvent immediately before its administration.
5. Dry, insoluble products which are combined with a suitable vehicle just before its administration.

The above mentioned preparations may be administered by any of the routes such as subcutaneous, intradermal, intramuscular, intravenous, intraspinal, intracisternal, intrathecal, intracardiac, or intraarticular. Out of these routes, the subcutaneous, intramuscular and intravenous are the most commonly used routes of injections for the administration of drugs, but the nature of the product will determine the particular route of administration which may be employed. For example, in case of intravenous injections, the drug in an aqueous solution is introduced directly into the vein whereas suspensions would not be introduced directly into the blood stream, because the insoluble particles of suspensions may block the capillaries. Subcutaneous injection should contain water soluble and non-irritating drugs and should be isotonic with body fluids to avoid irritation and pain. For intramuscular injection the drug may be dissolved or suspended in an aqueous or oily vehicle but the drugs dissolved in aqueous vehicles are absorbed faster than the drugs in oily solutions or suspensions in oily vehicle.

Essential Qualities of a Parenteral Product

A parenteral product must possess the following characteristics :

1. It should be free from living microorganisms and microbial products.
2. It should be free from pyrogens.
3. It should be free from foreign particles such as dust, fibres, etc.
4. It should be free from chemical contaminants.
5. It should be isotonic with body fluids.
6. It should have matching specific gravity with respect to some body fluids.
7. Multidose injections must contain preservatives.
8. Container/closure must not affect the product.

FORMULATION OF PARENTERAL PRODUCTS

In the development of parenteral products the pharmacist should have thorough knowledge and understanding of the principles involved and utmost care must be taken regarding accuracy, cleanliness and overall quality of the product. The medicinal substances used in the formulation of injections should be free from microbial and pyrogenic contamination. Whenever possible special parenteral grades of drugs which are commercially available should be used.

Only a minimum number of absolutely necessary additives in smallest possible quantities should be added. Excessive use of additives in parenteral products should be avoided since sometimes the metabolism of these additives becomes a problem. Some of the additives which are commonly used in the formulation of parenteral products are described below :

1. Vehicles

In the development of a parenteral product one will have to use a suitable vehicle for dissolving or suspending the medicaments. The most suitable vehicle for this purpose is water because aqueous preparations are tolerated well by the body and are the safest and easiest to administer. The water should be chemically pure and free from pyrogens. When water free from dissolved gases is required, it should be freshly boiled, cooled and stored in a well closed container to avoid reabsorption of oxygen and carbon dioxide.

Oily vehicles are used when the use of water is contraindicated in one way or the other, e.g., (a) when the medicament in insoluble or slightly soluble in water; (b) to increase the stability of the preparation; or (c) to prolong the duration of action of a drug. The commonly used fixed oils from vegetable origin are cottonseed oil, peanut oil, olive oil, sesame oil, etc. These oils should be free from rancid odour and taste. Mineral oils like liquid paraffin are rarely used since they are not absorbed from the tissues after injection.

Sometimes propylene glycol, polyethylene glycol and glycerin usually diluted with sterile water are used to prepare solutions for injections. They are used as solvents as well as to increase the stability of certain preparations.

Whenever non-aqueous vehicles are used for the preparation of injections, they must be administered by intramuscular injections only, accidental introduction by subcutaneous or intravenous injection may lead to serious results.

2. Added Substances

These substances are added to increase the stability or quality of the product and may include solubilising agents, antibacterial agents, antifungal agents, antioxidants, chelating agents, buffers, isotonicity factors, hydrolysis inhibitors, wetting, suspending and antifoaming agents, etc. These agents should be used only when it is absolutely necessary to use them and they must be used in the minimum possible quantity. These additives must be selected with great care so that they may not affect the entire formulation.

(a) Solubilising Agents

The solubilities of insoluble or poorly soluble drugs in water can be increased by co-solvents, complex formation or by adding surfactants like tweens, polysorbates, etc., which act by miceller solubilization.

(b) Stabilizers

Since oxidation and hydrolysis takes place more rapidly in drugs when they are in solution form therefore they must be suitably protected from oxidation and hydrolysis. To prevent oxidation either a suitable antioxidant is added or the product is sealed in an atmosphere of nitrogen or carbon dioxide so as to replace oxygen in the product thus minimising oxidation. Hydrolysis can be prevented either by replacing a part or whole of water in the preparation by a non-aqueous vehicle or by adjusting the pH of the preparation.

(c) Buffers

When the degradation of the preparation is due to change in pH it can be prevented by adding buffer systems which will maintain the necessary pH at desired level. Acetates, citrates and phosphates are the principal buffer systems used in this way.

(d) Antibacterial Agents

Bacteriostatic or fungistatic agents must be present in multidose containers. They must be added in adequate quantities to prevent the multiplication of microorganisms which may be accidentally introduced into the preparation while withdrawing a dose from the multidose containers. Among the compounds most frequently used as antibacterials agents are benzalkonium chloride 0.01%, phenol or cresol 0.5%, chlorocresol 0.2%, phenylmercuric nitrate 0.002% and chlorobutanol 0.5%. Care must be taken in selecting the antibacterial agent that it should be compatible with all other components of the formulation and should not be removed from solution by rubber closures of the package.

Bacteriostatic agents should not be used in single dose containers because the contents of these remain sterile until opened and the solution is injected but they may be included in those single dose containers which are to be sterilized by 'heating with a bactericide'.

(e) Isotonicity Factors

Parenteral preparations should be isotonic with blood serum or other body fluids to reduce irritation and pain of injection in areas with nerve endings. The isotonicity of a solution may be adjusted by adding sodium chloride, borax, etc., in suitable quantities but these materials should be non-toxic and must be compatible with other components of the formulation.

(f) Wetting, Suspending and Emulsifying Agents

In a parenteral suspension a wetting agent is used to reduce the interfacial energy between the solid particles and the liquid, so as to prevent the formation of lumps. They also act as antifoaming agents to subside the foam produced during shaking of the preparation. The wetting agents commonly used are tween 80 and sorbitan trioleate. The suspending agents generally used are methyl cellulose, carboxymethyl cellulose, acacia and gelatin.

Emulsifying agents are used in sterile emulsions. For this purpose lecithin is generally used. Gelatin may be added to aqueous vehicles to prolong the effect of the drug.

GENERAL PROCEDURE OF PREPARATION OF INJECTIONS

It is the general requirement that all the parenteral products must be free from foreign particles and micro-organisms. To achieve this aim care must be taken regarding the cleanliness and sterilization of area, atmosphere, persons involved and the materials used in the preparation of injections.

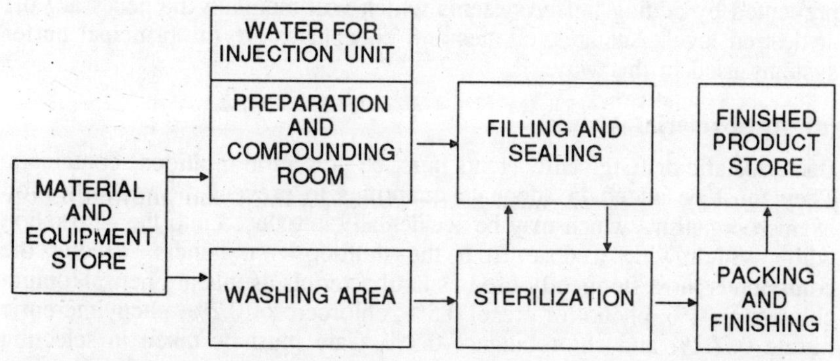

Fig. 12.2 Flow diagram for the manufacture of parenteral products.

The area and atmosphere of the room where the process is to be carried out must be free from dust, fibres and micro-organisms. This can be achieved with laminar flow system and by disinfectants. All the equipments which are likely to come in contact with the preparation must be thoroughly cleaned and sterilized. The workers should be highly trained and skilled. They should wear sterilized special clothings including hoods and gloves. They should take all sorts of precautions to avoid contamination because even the entry of a single microbe can render the product useless and harmful.

Parenteral preparations should be prepared from substances of the highest purity which have been accurately weighed and dissolved in pyrogen free distilled water or any other suitable solvent. Utmost care must be taken regarding the cleanliness in all operations. The solution so formed is passed through different grades of filters to remove foreign particles. The filters may be made from sintered glass, asbestos porcelain, etc. Now a days membrane filters composed of cellulose ester or polycarbonate are commonly used for filtering the parenteral solutions. Bacteria-proof filters are used to remove bacterias from the solutions.

After the preparation and suitable filtration of the solution it is packaged in suitable containers like ampoules, vials or bottles. Before filling the solution into these containers they must be thoroughly cleaned, dried and sterilized. The closures used should be of very high quality and must be sterilized.

On small scale, filling can be carried out with the help of hypodermic syringes attached with long needles, burettes, etc. The sealing of the ampoules can be done by fusion of glass in hot flames of blast burner or blow torch burner specially designed for this purpose. But now a days filling and sealing is done on very sophisticated automatic machines.

After filling and sealing the containers they are sterilized by means of dry heat or moist heat. For dry heat sterilization hot air ovens are used whereas for moist heat sterilization autoclaves are used. Oily and non-aqueous preparations must be sterilized by dry heat at a temperature of 160°C for two hours or at 170°C for one hour. Thermostable aqueous solutions should be sterilized by steam under pressure in autoclave at a temperature of 121°C for 20 minutes. Whereas aqueous solutions of thermolabile drugs cannot be sterilized by autoclaving therefore they must be passed through bacteria-proof filters to remove microbes.

After the filled containers have been sterilized and allowed to cool, they are inspected for clarity. Those containers which pass the clarity test are properly labelled and packaged into final containers.

PRECAUTIONS FOR ASEPTIC WORK TO PREVENT CONTAMINATION

1. As far as possible minimum number of persons should work in the injection department. Lesser the number of persons in the department, less will be the chances of contamination.
2. Persons trained in aseptic techniques should be allowed to work in the injection department.
3. Before entering the sterile area they must wash their hands which should then be treated with antiseptic solution, wear gloves, dress changed, hair covered, wear face mask and a hood over the head. The garments worn must not shed fibres and other particles.
4. The air in the processing area must be free from contaminants which is done by fitting a laminar air flow in the area.
5. Ultraviolet lamps should be fitted above the doors, working tables and room ceilings.
6. Walls should be painted in such a way that they can be easily cleaned, washed and disinfected.
7. There should be minimum hide-outs.
8. Furniture used should be minimum and they should be fitted with stainless steel or sunmica tops and other surfaces.

9. Double door entry should be provided. There should be minimum number of windows which should be of glazed panels. The windows may be kept closed.
10. Equipment is the major source of contamination, therefore, it must be thoroughly cleaned before and after its use. Wherever possible sterilized equipment should be used.
11. Frequent tests should be performed in the aseptic area to check the maintenance of sterility.
12. Whenever contamination is detected, its source should be identified and suitable methods adopted to check contamination.

MANUFACTURING OF PARENTERAL PREPARATIONS

Following steps are involved in the manufacturing of parenteral preparations :

1. Washing and cleaning of containers, closures and equipment.
2. Collection of materials.
3. Compounding the preparation.
4. Filtration.
5. Distributing the preparation in final containers.
6. Sealing the containers.
7. Sterilization.
8. Labelling and packaging.
9. Evaluation of parenteral preparations.

1. Washing and Cleaning of Containers, Closures and Equipment

All the containers, closures, and glass equipments required in parenteral preparations are thoroughly cleaned with detergent then washing with free flowing water followed by rinsing it with water for injection. As far as possible the various components of the apparatus should be separated and then cleaned. For small number of items washing can be done manually but on large scale automatic washing machines are used. High speed bottle brushes and multijet rinsers are used for this purpose. Finally, they are dried and sterilized by suitable methods.

2. Collection of Materials

The various materials required for the formulation of parenteral preparations are weighed and collected in the preparation room. All the ingredients, i.e., the medicaments, vehicles and additives used should be of the highest purity. Whenever water is to be used as vehicle, water free from pyrogens must be used.

3. Compounding the Preparation

For mixing and compounding a set procedure must be followed. Before mixing, the formulator must decide the order of mixing and he should have clear picture in his mind that what type of preparation will be obtained, i.e., regarding its colour, viscosity, etc.

4. Filtration

The solutions so formed are then passed through a suitable filter media to remove all the foreign particles. If the solutions are required to be sterilized by means of bacteria-proof filters then they are passed through suitable bacteria-proof filter. For this purpose sintered glass, asbestos or porcelain filters are used. Now a days membrane filters composed of cellulose ester or polycarbonate are commonly used for filtering the parenteral solutions.

5. Distributing the Preparation in Final Containers

After filtration and sterilization the solutions are distributed into final containers like ampoules, vials and bottles which are previously cleaned and sterilized. Ampoules are used for filling single doses whereas vials are used for filling multidoses. Bottles are generally used for filling transfusion fluids. On small scale filling can be carried out manually with the help of hypodermic syringes attached with long needles, burettes, etc. On large scale automatic filling machines are used. About 300 or more containers per minute can be filled with these machines.

Powders are little difficult to fill as compared to liquids. On small scale, solids like antibiotics are divided by weighing and then filled into individual containers or approximate quantity of the powdered drug can be filled in the container which is finally weighed on a balance. On large scale filling of powders is done by machines.

At the time of filling the ampoules, care should be taken that the solution should not touch the neck of the ampoule and it should be filled below the constriction of the neck of the ampoule otherwise it may lead to different problems such as cracking and staining at the time of sealing the ampoules.

6. Sealing the Containers

Sealing of the containers should be done as soon as possible to prevent the contamination of the contents. The rubber closures are fitted on the vials and bottles and sealed by crimping the aluminium caps which may be done manually or by mechanical means.

On small scale the ampoules are sealed manually by rotating the neck of the ampoule in the flame of bunsen burner or blast burner to soften the glass which ultimately fuses to close the ampoule. This is known as tip sealing but this is not a sure method of sealing because leakage generally occurs. Another method is that the neck of the ampoule is constantly rotated in the bunsen flame and when the glass softens, the tip is held firmly with a forceps or any other device and pulled quickly away from the body of the ampoule which is still rotated. A small capillary tube is formed which is closed by twisting. This method is known as pull sealing.

Although this is a slow process but the seals are more perfect than tip sealing.

7. Sterilization

Depending on the nature of products they may be sterilized by any suitable method.

Thermostable preparations are sterilized by autoclaving at a temperature of 115°C for 30 minutes or at 121°C for 20 minutes. Oily injections can be sterilized by hot air ovens at 160°C for 2 hours or at 170°C for one hour.

Thermolabile preparations are sterilized by passing through suitable bacteria-proof filters or by means of chemicals.

8. Labelling and Packaging

All the containers, i.e., ampoules, vials and bottles should be properly labelled with name of the preparation, quantity, batch number, lot number, date of manufacture, date of expiry (if any), storage conditions, retail price and manufacturer's address.

The labelled containers should be packaged in cardboard or plastic containers so that there is no breakage during transportation or handling. Ampoules should be packed in partitioned boxes.

Intravenous Fluids (Large Volume Parenterals)

Large volume of parenteral solutions are generally administered by intravenous infusion to supply body fluids, electrolytes or to provide nutrition to the body. They are administered in volumes of 250 ml to a number of litres per day by slow intravenous drip. Especial precautions must be taken that the solutions are free from foreign particles and they should be isotonic with body fluids.

It is essential that large volume 1/v injections and fluids are free from pyrogens as the injection of large amounts of these solutions may cause extremely serious thermal reactions in the patient. Since large volume of intravenous fluids are administered at a time so these solutions may not contain bacteriostatic agents or other additives. They are packaged in large single-dose glass or plastic containers.

Common examples of large volume parenterals which are generally used include :

1. Dextrose injection

It contains 2.5, 5, 10, 20% or other concentrations of dextrose. This solution is used as fluid and nutrient replenisher.

2. Dextrose and sodium chloride injection

It contains dextrose from 2.5 to 25% and sodium chloride from 0.11 to 0.9%. This solution is used as fluid, nutrient and electrolyte replenisher.

3. Fructose injection

It contains 10% fructose and is used as fluid replenisher and nutrient.

4. Fructose and sodium chloride injection

It contains 10% fructose and 0.9% sodium chloride. This solution is used as fluid, nutrient and electrolyte replenisher.

5. Mannitol injection

It contains 5, 10, 15, 20 and 25% mannitol and is used as diagnostic aid in renal function determinations and diuretic.

6. Mannitol and sodium chloride injection

It contains 5, 10 and 15% mannitol and 0.45% sodium chloride and is used as diuretic.

7. Ringer's injection

It contains 0.86% sodium chloride, 0.03% potassium chloride and 0.033% calcium chloride. This solution is used as fluid and electrolytic replenisher.

8. Lactated Ringer's injection

It contains 2-7 mEq. calcium, 4 mEq. potassium, 130 mEq. sodium and 2.45 gm lactate per litre. This solution is used as systemic alkalizer, fluid and electrolytic replenisher.

9. Sodium chloride injection

It is also known as normal saline solution and contains 0.9% sodium chloride. This solution is used as fluid and electrolyte replenisher and isotonic vehicle.

The above mentioned intravenous fluids are used in maintenance therapy for the patients who are to undergo surgery or have undergone surgery, or for unconscious patients who are unable to take fluids, electrolytes and nutrition orally. These solutions may also be used in replacement therapy in those patients who have suffered a heavy loss of fluids and electrolytes as in the case of severe diarrhoea or vomiting.

Parenteral Hyperalimentation (Total Parenteral Nutrition, TPN)

This is the infusion of large volumes of basic nutrients which are sufficient to produce active tissue synthesis and growth. These solutions contain high concentrations of dextrose (about 20%), electrolytes, vitamins and proteins. These solutions are administered slowly through a large vein and near to the heart for rapid dilution of the concentrated hyperalimentation fluid so as to minimize the risk of tissue or cellular damage due to hypertonicity of the solution.

Effect of incorporating drugs to infusion bottles

It is the general practice of nurses that certain drugs like antibiotics, vitamins, etc., are frequently incorporated into large volume parenterals by injecting the drug through the rubber closure into the bottles of infusion fluids. This practice is very dangerous because it may lead to :

1. Bacterial growth as no infusion contains a bactericide rather sugars present in infusions provide good medium for bacterial growth.
2. The added drugs may lead to interaction between the drugs and additives which may result in certain visible changes such as haziness, precipitation, crystallization, discolouration, etc., or may affect the efficacy or potency of the therapeutic agent which is not desirable.

It is the responsibility of the pharmacist to have thorough knowledge about the physical and chemical compatibility of the additives in the solution in which it is placed. He should discourage addition of medicaments to bottles of infusion fluids and suggest some suitable means of administering additional intravenous drugs.

Marketed Injections

1. Calmpose injection (Ranbaxy Labs Ltd., New Delhi - 110019).
2. Fortwin injection (Ranbaxy Labs Ltd., New Delhi - 110019).
3. Chloromycetin 1/m injection [Parke-Davis (India) Ltd., Bombay - 400021].
4. Terramycin 1/m injection (Pfizer Ltd., Bombay - 400021).
5. Aminophylline injection [Rathi Labs (Hindustan) Pvt. Ltd., Patna - 800013].
6. Atropine sulphate injection [Rathi Labs (Hindustan) Pvt. Ltd., Patna - 800013].
7. Calcium gluconate injection [Rathi Labs (Hindustan) Pvt. Ltd., Patna - 800013].
8. Compound sodium chloride injection [Rathi Labs (Hindustan) Pvt. Ltd., Patna - 800013].
9. Calcium-Sandoz 10% injection [Sandoz (India) Ltd., Bombay - 400018].
10. Benzyl penicillin G sodium injection (Sarabhai Chemicals, Vadodra - 390007).

Irrigation and Dialysis Solutions

Irrigation and dialysis solutions are quite similar to parenteral solutions as they are subjected to same standards. The difference is in their use. These solutions are not injected into the vein but are used outside the circulatory system. Since these types of solutions are generally used in large volumes so they are packed in large volume plastic containers.

Irrigation solutions are used for bathing or washing the wounds, surgical incisions or body tissues. A large number of official and patent irrigation solutions are available in the market. Some of them include Ringer's irrigation USP, sodium chloride irrigation USP, sterile water for irrigation USP.

Dialysis Solutions

Dialysis may be defined as the process by which the substances are separated from one another due to their difference in diffusibility through membranes. The solutions used in dialysis are known as dialysis solutions. In cases of poisoning or kidney failure or in cases where kidney transplantation is to be done, dialysis is an emergency life-saving procedure. In the case of renal failure, the removal of waste products and the maintenance of electrolyte balance is done either by haemodialysis or intraperitoneal dialysis.

1. Haemodialysis

Haemodialysis is used to remove toxins from the blood. In this method blood from a convenient artery is shunted through a polyethylene catheter through an artificial dialyzing membrane bathed in dialyzing fluid. The dialyzing membrane is permeable to urea, electrolytes and dextrose but not to plasma proteins and lipids. Substances such as urea which are in excess in the blood pass out in the fluid. After the dialysis the blood is freed from air bubbles and clots and is returned back to the body circulation through a suitable vein.

The fluids used in the artificial kidney are called haemodialysis solutions. Large quantities of such solutions are used daily in kidney units of the hospitals and it is not possible to handle such a large volumes. This problem is solved by preparing 35 × or 40 × strong solutions which are diluted afterwards.

Labelling

The concentrated haemodialysis solutions must be labelled with :

(i) The name of the solution, e.g., concentrated haemodialysis solution (35 × or 40 × as the case may be).
(ii) The strength of each ingredient.
(iii) The batch number.
(iv) Instructions regarding its dilution.
(v) Storage conditions.

2. Intraperitoneal Dialysis

In this technique the peritoneal cavity is irrigated with the dialysis solution and the peritonium acts as the semi-permeable membrane thereby the toxic substances normally excreted by the kidney are removed. A number of dialysis solutions are commercially available which contain dextrose, vitamins, minerals, electrolytes and amino acids. The solutions are made hypertonic to plasma to avoid absorption of water from the dialysis solution into the circulation. The intraperitoneal dialysis solutions must be sterile and should be free from pyrogens. These solutions are similar in composition to haemodialysis solutions except in the following respects :

(i) Because these solutions are ready for use so they are in very dilute form.
(ii) They always contain calcium and magnesium ions.
(iii) They do not contain any potassium ions if the need arises then potassium chloride is administered separately.
(iv) In these solutions anhydrous dextrose is used whereas in haemodialysis solutions dextrose (monohydrate) is used because such solutions are not injected.
(v) In these solutions the solvent used is water for injection.

Labelling

(i) The name of the solution, e.g., peritoneal dialysis solution.
(ii) The strength of each ingredient.
(iii) The batch number.
(iv) The volume in the container.
(v) The instructions that the solution is not for intravenous use.
(vi) An instruction to discard the unused part of the solution.

Evaluation of Parenteral Preparations

In the preparation of parenteral products strict quality control tests must be carried out throughout the entire process of preparation of a parenteral product to give assurance that the final product meets the required standards. Raw materials must be subjected to quality and pyrogen tests. Various tests, readings and observations must be made during the process to assure that the specifications are being met. Various tests and assays should be performed on the finished preparation to ensure that it meets the required specifications. In addition to the usual chemical and biological tests the following tests should be carried out on the parenteral preparations for their standardization.

(a) Sterility test.
(b) Pyrogen test.
(c) Clarity test.
(d) Leaker test.

(a) Sterility Test

Since all parenteral preparations are required to be sterile, they should be tested for sterility and must comply with the official test for sterility described in U.S.P. These tests are performed on all lots of injections in their final containers. The samples may be taken at random to represent the entire lot of the preparation. Hence the word 'Lot' for sterility testing means that group of product containers which has been subjected to same sterilization procedures.

According to U.S.P. there are two basic methods for sterility testing : (a) Direct inoculation of test samples on culture media; (b) Filtration technique.

In the direct inoculation method an aliquot quantity of the material under test is transferred to culture tubes containing a measured volume of a suitable culture medium like fluid Thioglycolate Medium or Thioglycolate Broth Medium. This whole operation, i.e., opening the containers, taking aliquot quantity of the material under test and transferring it to the culture medium contained in the tubes must be carried out under aseptic conditions and every precaution must be taken to prevent the accidental entry of micro-organisms into the test. These tubes are plugged with sterilized cotton wool and incubated for seven days at a temperature of 30 to 35°C. Positive and negative control tubes containing the culture media must be incubated under same conditions to confirm sterility and growth promoting properties of the medium. The material under test is considered sterile if there is no growth of micro-organisms in the tubes but if there is any turbidity or growth then the test must be repeated 2nd time with fresh sample of material and culture medium because in the first test the bacterial growth may be due to accidental entry of micro-organisms. If the 2nd test also shows the growth it may be repeated 3rd time very carefully and if this time also growth appears then the material fails to pass the sterility test.

If the product has antimicrobial properties they must be neutralized or eliminated by dilution. For solids or oily materials which make the culture medium turbid and make it difficult to conclude whether the turbidity is due to microbial growth or due to material itself, the normal test may have to be modified by subculturing the medium. If turbidity in subculture does not appear the material is sterile but if turbidity appears it is due to microbial growth which shows that the material is not sterile.

(b) Pyrogen Testing

Pyrogens

Pyrogens are the metabolic products of micro-organisms and are produced by all micro-organisms, i.e., gram-negative, gram-positive and fungi, but gram-negative bacterias generally produce most potent pyrogenic substances. They are soluble, filterable, thermostable and non-volatile substances. Chemically they are lipid in nature, sometimes containing phosphorus and are usually attached to polysaccharide or an amino acid carrier.

When introduced in human beings they cause febrile reactions which include chills and fever with headache and pain in the back and legs. Pyrogens are rarely fatal but they produce significant discomfort to the patient.

The major source of pyrogens in parenteral preparations is the water used for the preparation of injections which can be rendered free from pyrogens by proper distillation of water and storing the water under suitable conditions which does not allow the bacterial contamination to take place. Other solvents and chemicals used in the preparation are another source of pyrogens. Antibiotics produced by fermentation process generally contain pyrogens which must be effectively removed from pharmaceutical preparations containing these antibiotics. Containers and equipments used in the process may be another source of pyrogens which can be washed thoroughly with apyrogenic water to reduce the pyrogenic contents. They can be sterilized by keeping in hot air oven at a temperature of 175°C for 3 to 4 hours. Pyrogens can be destroyed by heating in an autoclave in the presence of an acid, alkali or oxidising agent. They can be removed by adsorbing on some adsorbing agent like activated charcoal, asbestos pads or aluminium hydroxide gel but this method is not suitable for pharmaceutical preparations because some of the drugs may also be adsorbed with the pyrogens. It is better to prevent the introduction of pyrogens than an attempt to remove them.

(c) Pyrogen Test

Pyrogen tests are performed on all aqueous parenteral preparations. In this test rabbits are used as test animals because they show similar physiological response to pyrogenic substances like that of man but the rabbits are very sensitive to external stimuli, therefore they must be handled very carefully. Only the healthy and mature rabbits should be used.

The test is made by introducing a suitable quantity of the sample to be tested into the ear vein of the rabbit. Rectal temperature is noted at 1, 2 and 3 hours after the introduction of the injection. If there is any rise in temperature of 0.6° or more above the normal temperature which has been taken before giving the injection, then the test is considered positive and the preparation contains pyrogens but if the rabbits do not show any rise in temperature then the product is considered free from pyrogens. Generally 5-8 rabbits are used for this test and average is calculated. Now a days number of specialized equipments are available for performing the pyrogen test.

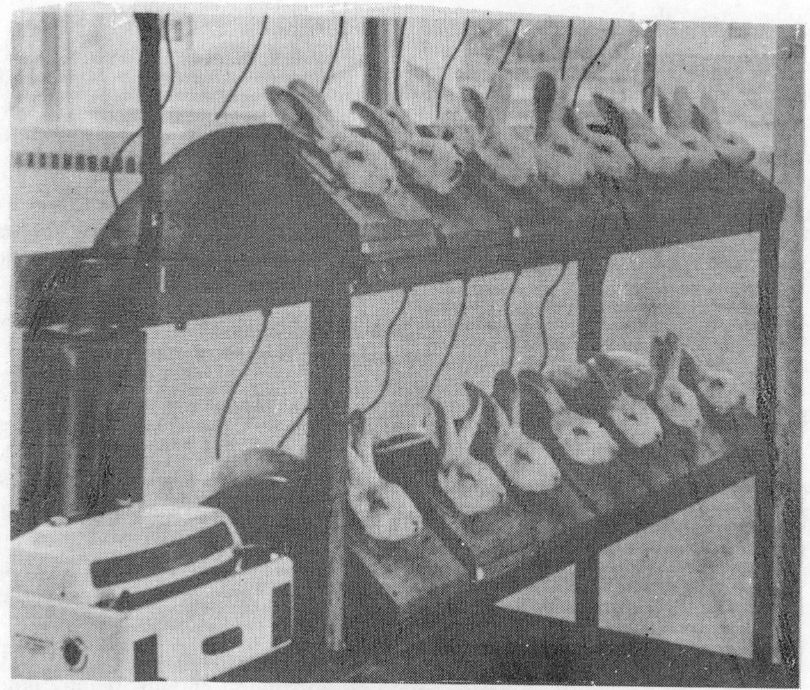

Fig. 12.3 Pyrogen testing.

(d) Clarity Test

The presence of particulate matter in parenteral preparations particularly those which are given intravenously are of serious concern. The particles larger than the size of red blood cells are dangerous, they may block the blood vessels with serious results. Therefore it is very necessary to check the final packages for clarity.

During the preparation of injections the particulate matter may enter from the environment including shedding from the body and clothes of persons, ceilings, walls and furniture of the room, from glass and rubber apparatus, the vehicles and the materials used. The particulate matter may also be introduced during administration if the infusion sets or syringes and needles are not properly cleaned and stored.

For checking the clarity of single dose or multidose packagings the unlabelled containers are held by the neck against strongly illuminated screen of which white surface is used for dark coloured particles and black surface for the detection of light coloured particles. The contents of the containers are slowly inverted and rotated and the solution examined for the presence of turbidity, dust or any other foreign particles. If any particulate matter is visible, the package is rejected. Certain instrumental methods have been developed and are widely used in the industries.

(e) Leaker Test

All the ampoules which have been sealed by fusion must be subjected to leaker test to check that there should not be any passage for leaking of the contents from the containers. This test is performed by dipping the ampoules in a deeply coloured dye solution for which 1% solution of methylene blue is used. The whole process is carried out in a vacuum chamber under negative pressure. When the vacuum is released the coloured solution will enter the ampoules with defective sealing. After careful washing of ampoules from outside, the dye can be seen in the leaker ampoules.

This test is not performed on vials and bottles because of flexibility of rubber, moreover the dye will badly stain the rubber stoppers.

ISOTONIC SOLUTIONS

All the ophthalmic and injectable solutions should be isotonic, e.g., ophthalmic solutions should be isotonic with lachrymal secretions (tears) to prevent irritation and pain, similarly, injectable solutions should be isotonic with blood plasma. Solutions having the same osmotic pressure are said to be isotonic. As compared to blood plasma if a solution has lower osmotic pressure it is said to be hypotonic but if it has higher osmotic pressure it is said to be hypertonic.

The solutions which are not isotonic with plasma may be harmful to use. On injecting the hypotonic solutions into blood stream, it may enter the red blood cells in an attempt to produce equilibrium. The cells swell rapidly until they burst leading to haemolysis. As this damage is irreversible it may lead to serious danger to red blood cells.

When hypertonic solution is injected into the blood stream, the water comes out of the membrane of red blood cells in order to reach equilibrium. The cells shrink leading to crenulation which is only a temporary damage. When the osmotic pressure of two solutions becomes equal the damaged cells will come to their original position. Hence hypertonic solutions may therefore be administered without permanent damage to the blood cells. They should be injected slowly to ensure rapid dilution into the blood stream and to minimise the crenulation of blood cells.

For the adjustment of tonicity of injectable solutions, substances like sodium chloride and dextrose, etc., are added. About 0.9% solution of sodium chloride is isotonic, 0.45 solution is hypotonic and 5% solution of sodium chloride is hypertonic with plasma.

Packaging of Parenteral Products

The packaging of parenteral preparations is an extremely important part of the product. The package must be neat and attractive in appearance so as to convey to the user the quality, purity and reliability of the product. The label on the package should be neat and clean and must provide the necessary information regarding identity, strength and for its use. Furthermore the package should protect the product from physical damage during transport, handling and storage. The light-sensitive products should be protected from ultraviolet rays.

Containers including closures for injectables must not interact physically or chemically with the preparation so as to alter its strength or effectiveness. The glass used for the preparation of containers must be of very high quality, clear, colourless or of a light amber colour so as to permit the inspection of its contents. Products sensitive to alkalies should be packed in neutral glass or in such glass containers which have passed the limit tests for alkalinity. Injections are generally packed either in single dose containers or in multi-dose containers.

Single-dose Container

A single dose container is a hermetically sealed container which contains only one dose of the sterile drug. When such container is once opened it cannot be re-sealed with assurance that sterility has been maintained. Commonly single dose injections are known as ampoules which are sealed by fusion of glass of the container under aseptic conditions.

Multi-dose Container

A multi-dose container contains a number of doses and are sealed in such a way that the rubber closures allow the withdrawal of doses by puncture with hypodermic needles, thus successive portions of the contents can be withdrawn without changing the strength, quality or purity of the remaining portion.

The closures used in multi-dose containers create many problems which must be taken care of before selecting the closure. The main problems are absorption of materials from the products and shedding of undesirable soluble or insoluble components to the preparation. Sometimes the closures react with the products.

Plastic containers are not very commonly used for packaging the injections. However the use of plastic containers is increasing day by day for packaging infusion and dialysing fluids and for blood. These types of containers have advantages over glass containers that they are unbreakable, light and disposable, occupy less storage space and easy to handle.

Some recent trends in packaging of parenteral products

Generally the parenteral products are packed in ampoules, multidose vials and transfusion bottles but numerous difficulties have been encountered with these types of containers. In ampoules the greatest difficulty is that when it is broken or cut to withdraw the dose, fragments of glass enter into the contents thus contaminate it with glass pieces. In the case of vials and transfusion bottles the problem may arise due to rubber closures. Therefore due to these problems some other types of packages have been designed.

A special kind of vial known as Mix-O-Vial marketed by Upjohn Company is used for packing either the sterile powders and their vehicles or for separating incompatible drugs. This vial has two compartments, the upper and the lower compartment. The lower chamber usually contains the dry ingredients and the upper one contains the liquid diluent or the vehicle. These two compartments are separated by a specially designed centre seal.

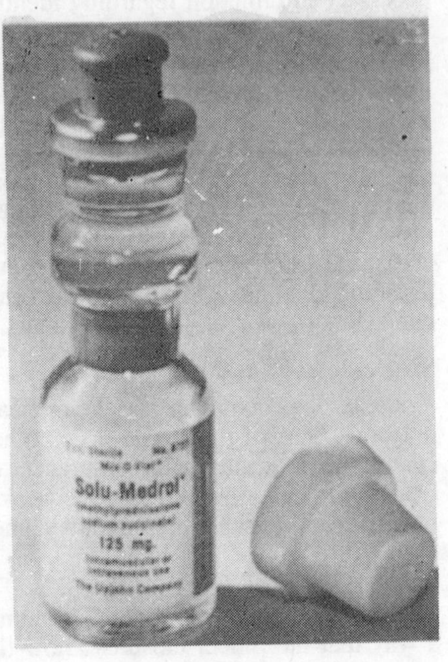

Fig. 12.4 Mix-O-Vial.

For using the vial, the uppermost dust cover is removed, pressure is applied to the top plunger with the help of thumb which dislodges the centre seal and allows the liquid to blow in the lower chamber. The vial is shaken until a solution is obtained. Then the solution is withdrawn by inserting a syringe needle. These types of vials have advantages that :

1. They offer stability to the product.
2. They are convenient.
3. They offer safety as the right drug will be mixed with proper diluent and in the correct proportions.

Prefilled disposable syringes are another recent technique for packaging the parenteral products. Now a days a variety of prefilled disposable syringes are marketed under proprietary names such as 'Abboject' (Abbot), 'Isoject' (Pfizer), 'U-ject' (Upjohn), etc.

Marketed mix-o-vial preparation by Upjohn Company, Kalamzoo M-49001, USA.

Solu-Medrol sterile powder

Contains :

Methylprednisolone sodium succinate for injection USP 1 gram for intramuscular or intravenous use.

Revision Questions

I. Very short answer type questions :

(A) Define the following :

(i) Parenteral preparations
(ii) Water for injection
(iii) Intravenous fluids
(iv) Dialysis solutions
(v) Pyrogens

(B) Fill in the blanks :

(i) Parenteral preparations should be ...... through the same route for which they are ....
(ii) Multidose injections ...... preservatives.
(iii) The air in the processing area is made free from contaminants by fitting ...... in the area.
(iv) Persons working in the manufacturing of injectables must wear ...... and ....
(v) TPN stands for ....
(vi) Haemodialysis is done to remove ...... from the blood.
(vii) Clarity test is done to ensure that the parenteral product is free form ....

(C) Answer the following questions in brief :

(i) Name different types of parenteral preparations.
(ii) Name different types of vehicles used in the preparation of parenteral products.
(iii) Name various tests which are to be performed for the evaluation of parenteral products.
(iv) Name different types of adjuvants used in the formulation of parenteral preparations.
(v) Give a flow diagram for the manufacture of parenteral products.
(vi) Name the steps involved in the manufacture of parenteral preparations.

II. Short answer type questions

1. Discuss the advantages and disadvantages of parenteral products.
2. Explain the essential qualities of parenteral products.
3. What is aseptic work? Discuss the precautions which must be followed during aseptic work.
4. Describe the recent trends in packaging of parenteral products along with suitable diagram.
5. Write short notes on the following :
   (i) Precautions to be taken during aseptic work.

(ii) Intravenous fluids.
(iii) Parenteral Hyper Alimentation (Total Parenteral Nutrition)
(iv) Effect of incorporating drugs to infusion bottles.
(v) Haemodialysis
(vi) Stability test
(vii) Pyrogen testing
(viii) Isotonic solutions.
(ix) Packing of parenteral products.
(x) Recent trends in packing of parenteral products.

III. Long answer type questions

1. What are "parenteral preparations"? Describe their advantages and disadvantages; also explain the essential qualities of a parenteral product.
2. What do you understand from the term 'route of administration'? Discuss various routes of administration of parenteral products.
3. Define the term ' parenteral products'. Discuss various additives used in the formulation of parenteral products.
4. Explain the term ' parenteral preparations' Describe various steps involved during manufacturing of parenteral preparations.
5. What is 'dialysis'? Describe different types of dialysis and fluids used in these dialysis.
6. Describe in brief the tests performed in the evaluation of parenteral products.
7. Discuss why is it necessary to perform evaluation tests for parenteral products? Explain pyrogen testing and clarity testing in detail.

Answers

I. (B)
(i) Introduced, meant for
(ii) Must contain
(iii) Laminar air flow
(iv) Gloves, hoods
(v) Total Parenteral Nutrition
(vi) Toxins
(vii) Foreign particles

13

Ophthalmic Products

These are the products which are to be instilled into the eye in the space between the eye lids and the eye balls. They may also be injected into various regions of the eye. Though they are not parenterals by definition but have many similar and often identical characteristics.

Ophthalmic preparations must be sterile and are prepared under the same conditions and by the same methods as other parenteral preparations. Solutions used during surgery must be sterile and should not contain any preservative. They should be supplied in single-use containers and any solution remaining at the end of the operation must be discarded. Since the capacity of the eye to retain liquid and ointment preparations is limited so they are generally administered in small volumes.

Types of Ophthalmic Products

Various ophthalmic products include :

1. Eye drops
2. Eye lotions
3. Eye suspensions
4. Contact lens solutions
5. Eye ointments
6. Ophthalmic inserts.

1. Eye Drops

Eye drops are sterile aqueous or oily solutions or suspensions for instillation into the eye. They are usually applied into the space between the eyeball and eyelids or on to the corneal surface. The main requirement of eye drops is that they should be sterile, usually isotonic, buffered and free from foreign particles to avoid irritation to the eye. They usually contain substances having antiseptic, anaesthetic, anti-inflammatory, mydriatic or miotic properties or substances used for diagnostic purposes.

Most of the eye drops contain aqueous vehicles rather than oily vehicles. Aqueous eye drops may support bacterial and fungal growth therefore these must be preserved by adding a suitable preservative for which purpose phenylmercuric nitrate or acetate 0.002%, benzalkonium chloride 0.01% and chlorhexidine acetate 0.01% may be used. Phenylmercuric nitrate should not be used in eye drops which are intended for prolonged treatment and benzalkonium chloride is not suitable as preservative for eye drops containing local anaesthetics.

The eye drops must be protected from contamination during use and must be used within two weeks after first opening of the container. Due to this reason eye drops should be prescribed in small amount, i.e., 5 to 10 ml for a limited number of applications. If larger volumes are prescribed they must be dispensed in a number of smaller containers rather than in one large container.

Eye drops should be dispensed in glass or suitable plastic containers with a screw cap fitted with a rubber teat and glass dropper for easy application of the drops or the containers may be fitted with a narrow nozzle from which the drops can be directly instilled into the eye. While using, care must be taken to avoid contamination by touching to the eyes or to the nozzle of the container. If this precaution is not taken the remaining solution may be contaminated and become unfit for use. In the hospital ward or out-patient departments, eye drops should not be used after one week after first opening of the container and in the operation theatre a new unopened container should be used for each patient.

Marketed Eye Drops

1. Albucid eye drops (Nicholas Labs. India Ltd., Bombay - 400088).

   Contains :

   Sulphacetamide sodium (i) 10%, (ii) 20%, (iii) 30%.

2. Betnisol eye/ear drops (Glaxo India Ltd., Bombay - 400025).

   Contains :

   Betamethasone sodium phos. 0.1%

3. Cortola-M eye drops (East India Pharmaceutical Works Ltd., Calcutta - 700071).

   Contains :

Sulphacetamide sodium	10%	W/V
Hydrocortisone acetate	1%	W/V
Phenylethyl alcohol	0.5%	

4. Enteromycetin eye drops (Dey's Medical Stores, Calcutta - 700087).

   Contains :

Chloramphenicol	0.5%
Phenyl mercuric nitrate	0.002%

5. Itone eye drops (Dey's Medical Stores, Calcutta - 700087).
6. Optacid eye drops (Dey's Medical Stores, Calcutta - 700087).

Contains :

Sulphacetamide sodium (i) 10%, (ii) 20%.

7. Locula eye drops (East India Pharmaceutical Works Ltd., Calcutta - 700071).

   Contains :

   Sod. sulphacetamide solu. (i) 10%, (ii) 20%, (iii) 30%.

8. Sofracort eye/ear drops (Roussel India Ltd., Bombay - 400018).
9. Soframycin eye drops (Roussel India Ltd., Bombay - 400018).

   Contains :

Framycetin sulph	5 mg
Phenylmercuric nitrate	0.002% W/V

2. Eye Lotions

Eye lotions or eye washes are sterile aqueous solutions used for irrigating the eye. Sodium chloride eye lotion is used to remove foreign substances from the eye. They are usually applied with a clean eye-bath or sterile fabric dressing and a large volume of solution is allowed to flow quickly over the eye.

Eye lotions are usually supplied in concentrated form and are required to be diluted with an equal volume of warm water immediately before use. They should be freshly prepared and should not be stored for more than 2-3 days as they may be contaminated with microorganisms on prolonged storage. Eye lotions should be isotonic and free from foreign particles to avoid irritation to the eye. The drugs used for preparing eye solutions include sodium chloride, sodium bicarbonate, boric acid, borax or zinc sulphate.

3. Eye Suspensions

Eye suspensions are not commonly used as compared to eye drops. They are only prepared when the drug is insoluble in the desired vehicle or unstable in solution form. They are also used to produce the sustained action of the preparation. Eye suspensions should have the following characteristics :

1. They should be sterile.
2. They should be isotonic, buffered and suitably preserved.
3. They should be of the desired viscosity.
4. They should be packaged in dropper type containers.
5. The particle size of the suspension should be non-irritating to the eyes.
6. The suspended particles must not agglomerate into large ones on storage.

7. The suspensions must be thoroughly shaken before each application to distribute the particles uniformly throughout the vehicle.

Examples of ophthalmic suspensions include :

(i) Dexamethasone ophthalmic suspension.
(ii) Hydrocortisone ophthalmic suspension.
(iii) Tetracycline hydrochloride ophthalmic suspension.

4. Contact Lens Solutions

Contact lenses are generally made from hard hydrophobic plastic known as polymethyl methacrylate but now a days some softer hydrophobic lenses are also used.

The wearers of hard contact lenses generally use two types of solutions.

(a) One before inserting the lenses into the eyes which is known as wetting solution.
(b) The other one used for overnight cleaning, soaking and storage which is known as storage solution.

(a) Wetting Solutions

Because of the hydrophobic nature of the polymethyl methacrylate it is poorly wetted by the lacrymal fluid of the eye and requires moistening with a wetting agent to render the surface of the lens hydrophylic, make the insertion easy and comfortable.

Since the contact lens solutions are used daily and years together so they must be prepared very carefully and the ingredients used should be of highest quality. The formulation of contact lens solutions may include a wetting agent, buffering agent, a thickening agent, a substance for adjusting the osmotic pressure, a preservative and a vehicle. The vehicle used is generally purified water. Tap water is not suitable because the dissolved salts present in it may lead to irritation in the eye.

(b) Storage Solutions

The contact lenses must be cleaned after use. After removing from the eye they are cleaned with wetting solution and rinsed with purified water. Then they are stored in a soaking solution with the intention to continue the cleaning process and prevent dehydration.

The formulation of storage solutions generally contain :

(i) A non-ionic surface active agent which will help in cleaning the lenses.
(ii) A blend of preservatives to prevent the bacterial growth. The solution should be changed after every few days because the preservatives may be practically inactivated by the organic materials present in the form of debris.

The label of the contact lens solutions must contain the instructions that the solution should be protected from contamination and the storage solution should be frequently changed.

Marketed Contact Lens Solutions

1. Bausch & Lomb multipurpose solution (Bausch & Lomb India Ltd., 89-Nehru Palace, New Delhi - 110019).
2. Gel-Clens cleaning solution (Consol Products, Wadala, Bombay - 400031).
3. Gel-Soak (Consol Products, Wadala, Bombay - 400031).
4. Comfort drops (Gay Labs, Karnal Road Ind. Area, Delhi - 110033).
5. Rinsol (Gay Labs, Karnal Road Ind. Area, Delhi - 110033).
6. VFLEX cleansing solution (Venu Contact Lens Pvt. Ltd., New Delhi - 110005).

5. Eye Ointments

These ointments are meant for application to the eye. They should be sterile and free from irritation. The ointment base selected for an eye ointment must be non-irritating to the eye and must permit the diffusion of the drug throughout the secretions of the eye and must melt close to the body temperature.

For the preparation of eye ointments the eye ointment base B.P. is used. This base consists of :

Yellow soft paraffin	80%
Liquid paraffin	10%
Wool fat	10%

In the eye ointment base B.P. yellow soft paraffin is used. White soft paraffin is not used because it is prepared by bleaching the yellow soft paraffin and the bleaching agent may remain sticking to the base even after careful washing, which if instilled into the eye may lead to irritation.

The liquid paraffin is used because it reduces the viscosity of the base thus make it easier to expel from the tube and apply to the eye.

Wool fat is included because it ensures satisfactory emulsification of the solution and helps in the absorption of active ingredients.

For the preparation of base all the ingredients are melted together on water bath and filtered through a coarse filter paper kept in a heated funnel. It is then sterilized at 150°C for one hour, immediately stored in a container so as to exclude micro-organisms before use.

The eye ointments can be prepared by two methods : (a) trituration method; and (b) fusion method. These methods have already been described in detail under the chapter ointments.

The preparation of eye ointments must be carried out under aseptic conditions and packing must also be done in sterile containers which should keep the preparation sterile until whole of it is used up. For packaging the eye ointments, previously sterilized tin, aluminium or plastic collapsible tubes are used. Now a days eye applicaps are available which contain only one application of the preparation.

Advantages

Eye ointments have certain advantages over eye drops that in the case of ointments the ocular contact time is increased and studies have shown that the ocular contact time is two to four times greater in ointments than eye solutions thus prolonged action of the drug can be produced.

Disadvantages

Eye ointments have disadvantage that on application it produces blurred vision for a short time as the ointment melts and is spread across the lens.

Marketed Eye Ointments

1. Betnisol eye ointment (Glaxo India Ltd., Bombay - 400025).

   Contains :

   Betamethasone sod-phosphate 0.1%

2. Betnisol-N eye ointment (Glaxo India Ltd., Bombay - 400025).

   Contains :

   Betamethasone sod-phosphate 0.1%
   Neomycin sulphate 0.5%

3. Enteromycetin ophthalmic ointment (Dey's Medical Stores, Calcutta - 70008).

   Contains :

   Chloramphenicol 1%

4. Soframycin ophthalmic ointment (Roussel India Ltd., Bombay - 400018).

   Contains :

   Framycetin sulphate 0.5% W/W
   Phenylmercuric nitrate 0.001% W/W

5. Terramycin ophthalmic ointment (Pfizer Ltd., Bombay - 400021).
6. Tetracycline eye ointment (Bombay Drug House Pvt. Ltd., Bombay - 400101).

   Contains :

   Tetracycline HCl 1%

Marketed Eye Applicaps

1. Chlorocort applicaps [Parke-Davis (India) Ltd., Bombay - 400025]

Each contains :

Chloramphenicol 1%

Hydrocortisone acetate 0.5%

2. Chloromycetin applicaps [Parke-Davis (India) Ltd., Bombay - 400025].

Each contains :

Chloromycetin 1%

6. Ophthalmic Inserts

Ophthalmic inserts are the new drug delivery systems for administering the drugs to the eyes. These are designed in such a way that they release the drug at predetermined and predictable rates thus eliminating the frequent administration of the drugs by the patient, even he is saved from the botheration of administering the drug at night time. In this way the chances of missing the doses are decreased.

Generally the inserts are elliptical in shape having the dimensions 13.4 × 5.7 mm and 0.3 mm in thickness. They are sterile and do not contain any preservative. They are flexible in nature and consist of multilayered structures the innermost being the core containing the medicament. This structure is surrounded by a layer of copolymer through which the drug diffuses at a constant rate. The rate of diffusion of the drug depends on the composition of the polymer, thickness of the membrane and the solubility of the drug.

The Pilocarpine inserts have proved quite useful and effective in glaucoma therapy. It is allowed to release the drug at desired rates for about seven days after which it is removed and replaced with new ones

Revision Questions

I. Very short answer type questions

(A) Define the following :

(i) Ophthalmic products
(ii) Eye drops
(iii) Eye lotions
(iv) Eye suspensions
(v) Contact lens solutions
(vi) Eye ointments
(vii) Ophthalmic inserts

(B) Fill in the blanks :

(i) Ophthalmic products should be ...... with lachrymal secretions to avoid ...... and ....
(ii) Eye drops are to be instilled between ...... and ....

(iii) Eye lotions are supplied in ...... form and must be diluted with ...... water immediately before use.
(iv) Eye suspensions are also used to produce ...... action of the preparation.
(v) ...... soft paraffin is not used as a base for the preparation of ophthalmic ointments.

II. Short answer type questions

(A) Explain the following :
(i) Explain why ophthalmic products are dispensed in small containers?
(ii) Describe the essential qualities of eye drops.
(iii) Why white soft paraffin is not used in the preparation of ophthalmic ointments? Give suitable formula for ophthalmic ointment base.
(iv) Discuss the formulation of eye drops.
(v) What are eye ointments? Describe the advantages and disadvantages of eye ointments.

(B) Write short notes on the following :
(i) Ophthalmic products
(ii) Eye drops
(iii) Eye lotions
(iv) Eye suspensions
(v) Eye ointments
(vi) Contact lens solutions
(vii) Ophthalmic inserts

(C) Differentiate between the following :
(i) Eye drops and eye lotions
(ii) Eye lotions and contact lens solutions
(iii) Eye ointments and skin ointments

(D) Name at least three marketed preparations of :
(a) Eye drops
(b) Eye ointments

III. Long answer type questions

1. What are ophthalmic products? Name various ophthalmic products used. Describe the formulation of eye drops.
2. Define 'Contact lens solutions' describe various types of contact lens solutions in detail.
3. What are eye ointments? How do they differ skin ointments? Discuss the method of preparation of eye ointments

Answers

I. B

(i) Isotonic, irritation, pain

(ii) Eyelids and eye ball

(iii) Concentrated, warm

(iv) Sustained

(v) White

Reference Books

1. Remington's Pharmaceutical Sciences, Mack Publishing Company, Pennsylvania.
2. Dispensing of Medication, Formerly Husa's Pharmaceutical Dispensing, Mack Publishing Co., Easton, Pennsylvania.
3. The Theory and Practice of Industrial Pharmacy, Lea and Febiger, Philadelphia.
4. Cooper and Gunn's Dispensing for Pharmaceutical Students, Pitman Medical Publishing Co. Ltd., London.
5. Clinical Pharmacy : A Text For Dispensing Pharmacy, Jenkins, Sperandio and Latiolais, McGraw-Hill Book Company, London.
6. Mithal : Text Book of Pharmaceutical Formulations, Birla Institute of Technology and Science, Pilani.
7. Schroff : Professional Pharmacy, Part V, Vol. I, National Book Centre, Dr. Sundari Mohan Avenue, Calcutta - 14.
8. Schroff : Professional Pharmacy, Part V, Vol. II, Five Stars Enterprises, Dr. Sundari Mohan Avenue, Calcutta - 14.
9. The Pharmacopoeia of India.
10. National Formulary of India.
11. The British Pharmacopoeia.
12. British Pharmaceutical Codex.
13. The Pharmacopoeia of United States.
14. Extra Pharmacopoeia Martindale.
15. The Pharmacopoeia of U.S.S.R.

Index